The Psychology of Addiction

Contemporary Psychology Series: 10

The Psychology of Addiction

Mary McMurran

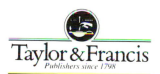

Taylor & Francis
Publishers since 1798

UK	Taylor & Francis Ltd, 4 John St., London WC1N 2ET
USA	Taylor & Francis Inc., 1900 Frost Road, Suite 101, Bristol, PA 19007

First published 1994

A Catalogue Record for this book is available from the British Library

ISBN 0 74840 0187 3
ISBN 0 74840 0188 1 (pbk)

Library of Congress Cataloging-in-Publication Data are available on request

Cover design by Amanda Barragry
Typeset in 11/13pt Garamond
by Graphicraft Typesetters Ltd., Hong Kong

Printed in Great Britain by Burgess Science Press, Basingstoke on paper which has a specified pH value on final paper manufacture of not less than 7.5 and is therefore 'acid free'.

For
Maureen Walker, my beloved sister;
Delia Cushway, my best friend; and
Gary Gilchrist, my favourite rock star.

Contents

List of Tables and Figures   viii

Series Editor's Preface   x

Preface   xiii

Chapter 1   Addiction: Misconduct and Disease   1

Chapter 2   Psychological Approaches to Addiction   31

Chapter 3   Initiation and Maintenance   51

Chapter 4   Dependence   73

Chapter 5   Change   97

Chapter 6   Prevention   131

Chapter 7   Postscript   159

References   161

Index   177

List of Tables and Figures

Figure 1.1	The balanced placebo design	26
Table 2.1	Factors that determine behaviour	32
Figure 2.1	The development of conditioned craving	35
Table 3.1	Prevalence of substance use by age	54
Table 3.2	Prevalence and amounts of drinking from a population census survey	54
Table 3.3	Cigarette smoking by gender	55
Table 3.4	Type of substance, frequency of use, and gender of user	55
Table 3.5	Deviant behaviours that occur in a cluster	62
Figure 3.1	The relationship among social factors, intrapersonal factors, expectations and alcohol use	66
Table 3.6	Stressful life events	67
Table 3.7	Risk factors for substance use in decreasing order of importance	67
Table 3.8	Risk factors for substance use	68
Table 4.1	Pay-off matrix	76
Table 4.2	Cues which elicit craving	91
Table 4.3	Capabilities required for self-control	92
Table 5.1	Therapist's tasks	102
Figure 5.1	Modules of intervention	103
Table 5.2	Self-motivational statements	105
Table 5.3	Techniques of motivational interviewing	106
Table 5.4	Methods of assessment	107
Figure 5.2	Self-monitoring diary	109
Table 5.5	Social skills programme	112
Table 5.6	Problem solving	114
Table 5.7	Muscle relaxation exercises	116
Table 5.8	Determinants of relapse	117

Table 5.9   Covert modelling script   119
Table 5.10   The Twelve Steps of Alcoholics Anonymous   129
Figure 6.1   A model of prevention of deviant behaviour   148
Table 6.1   Prevention programme   151

Series Editor's Preface

The following stories appeared in today's newspaper (*The Guardian*, Wednesday, 8th June, 1994): three tons of cocaine destined for the US were seized at an airstrip in Columbia; a lighthearted article on cannabis, pointing out that there are at least 1.5 million regular users of the drug in the UK; the Marquis of Blandford being placed on probation for eighteen months after pleading guilty to a series of theft and forgery offences, which had been committed largely as a result of his drug addiction; ten teenagers taken to hospital after overdosing on stolen drugs. These stories not only indicate the widespread use and fascination with the use of drugs in contemporary society, but also something more important. This is best illustrated by the last of these four stories, which concerns the ten youngsters in Durham, aged between fourteen and nineteen, who were taken to hospital after becoming violently sick following overdosing on drugs that had been stolen in a house burglary. Fortunately, most of the youngsters were released from hospital shortly after they were admitted, but at least one remained in a very serious condition. The stolen drugs that the youngsters ingested included Valium, methadone and Temazepam. It seems quite unlikely that the young people knew what these drugs were, or what their likely effects would be. However, they were quite happy, indeed paid money, to ingest or inject them into their bodies. One of those who overdosed was subsequently interviewed on the radio, and he said that using drugs was the only way of relieving the boredom of his life.

What is fascinating about this story (and also the story of the Marquis of Blandford) is the blind pursuit of altered states of consciousness without any care being taken as to the user's health or social well-being. If we add to the illicit substances that are the subject matter of Mary McMurran's book the other most commonly used drugs, namely alcohol, nicotine and caffeine, it is clear that the pursuit of drug induced changes in mental state is one of the few universals of human behaviour.

Looking back over history and across geographical locations, and across societies and cultures with all kinds of orientations, there seems to be almost always a central place for the use of drugs, especially by men. It is probably safe to say that for all of recorded history most people on this planet have used mind altering drugs in one form or another, and that a substantial proportion of users have been addicted. Often this addiction is socially accepted and, therefore, in one sense 'harmless', but often it results in socially unacceptable levels of dependence and is then, formally or informally, penalized. The point here is that using substances that alter brain processes is a normal part of human behaviour, indeed behaviour that those who are involved in it invest with a great deal of importance. The importance is marked by the willingness to pay substantial sums in money or in kind in order to obtain drugs, and to risk the personal and social effects that are contingent upon addiction.

The Durham youth who said that he used drugs in order to escape boredom was perhaps also revealing a near universal human truth. Now, my cat does not get bored I presume, but if it is in a state where there is not much to do it lies down in the sun or goes to sleep. This does not seem an option for many human beings. Our brains are constantly active while we are awake (and indeed while we sleep), and we need a certain level of stimulation in order to maintain a comfortable equilibrium. Where the level of stimulation required falls below the optimal, then there is either a search for increased stimulation, or the general level of arousal of the brain is damped down by taking some substance which alters its normal functioning. It has been suggested by eminent theorizers, such as Arthur Koestler, that the capacity for computing inherent in the human brain is too great for our own good, and leads to all kinds of personal and social problems. If we have more brain power than is needed for everyday functioning in our well ordered social world, then this additional power will find an outlet in non-essential activity, which may be socially valued (such as artistic endeavours), or socially devalued (such as the search for thrills, gratuitous violence, vandalism and drug use).

It is, therefore, necessary to approach drug use as a normal behaviour in which ordinary and well-adjusted people engage, as well as looking at the extreme end of the continuum of behaviour which results in severe personal addiction and social paralysis. Dr McMurran's book reviews the major psychological models of addiction and looks at the functions that addictions serve for those who suffer from them. It points out quite clearly that whether or not addictive behaviour is judged as problematic depends upon the circumstances and social context. It is clear that biological determinants of addiction play only a small role in the overall experience of the problem and, indeed in the case of many drugs, may be largely irrelevant. What the person who uses a drug expects to gain from its use and the consequences of that use is largely, if not entirely, socially determined.

Dr McMurran is one of Britain's leading experts on the role of drugs in the aetiology of criminal behaviour, and this expertise is evident throughout the book. The link between drugs and crime is, of course, a major concern of the media and the general public that often appears to be more important in the public mind than the use of the drugs themselves. Many of the attempts to introduce more stringent penalties for drug use are in fact indirect attempts to reduce the rate of criminal activity associated with the need to finance drug habits. I suspect that many people would be reasonably content to let addicts use their drug so long as they did not need to engage in all kinds of anti-social behaviour in order to be able to do so.

The final chapter is in some ways the most important as it tackles the very difficult topic of how to reduce the risk of addiction occurring. Prevention based upon disseminating knowledge does not work. This much is clear from many evaluation studies in health promotion. Even if people have all the information available about the harmfulness of certain substances or other behaviours, they will still engage in them if their motivation is strong enough. Dr McMurran suggests a model of prevention based upon inhibiting initiation and escalation by restricting access and changing the culture in which drug using occurs. In addition, she recommends a focus on harm minimization rather than complete prevention, which offers a more realistic chance of success, and is more likely to engage the experienced and inexperienced drug user alike in attempts at reducing the harmful effects of drugs in our society.

As with other books in this series, the reader will find this an accessible introduction to the concepts necessary to understand issues around drug use, and also will find, as they progress through the text, an increased familiarity with basic psychological concepts.

Ray Cochrane
Birmingham, June 1994

Preface

My favourite statement 'about the author' in any book I have read so far is in Jim Hankinson's *Bluff Your Way in Philosophy*. It says, 'At school he was widely held to be too clever by half; but these days, by dint of persistent intake of alcohol he is only too clever by about 10 per cent.' Being too clever by any degree was never one of my credentials, and does not explain how I came to write this book. I feel, however, that it is necessary to present some account of how I developed an interest in the subject of addiction and consequently came to write about it.

I have worked with offenders since 1980, first as a prison psychologist in a young offender centre, and more recently as a clinical psychologist in a secure psychiatric hospital. My main area of study over the years has been that of alcohol-related crime. I have made attempts to understand the link between drinking and offending, and to apply interventions to reduce both drinking and alcohol-related crime. My knowledge of addictive behaviours has, up to now, focused upon this one specific angle, and although I have written about alcohol and crime, I have not previously set out to summarize the psychological perspective on addictive behaviours. Writing this book presented me with the opportunity to broaden and clarify my own thoughts on the subject.

Another quotation comes to mind here. I have a book called *The Macmillan Treasury of Relevant Quotations*. A friend of mine once spotted this book on my shelf and asked the pertinent question 'Relevant to what'? One citation is relevant to the subject of this book. It is by Frederick Goodyear, who mentioned in his letters, 'It is really very curious that people get more muddled in their heads by thinking about intoxicants than by drinking them.' I do not actually know who Frederick Goodyear was, or to whom he was writing, but I think he has a point. In writing this book, I learned a great deal about the topic of addiction. Having to think about intoxicants forced me to defuzz my woolly thinking and straighten out my crooked logic. I hope that I have managed to make some sense of addiction for the reader.

Of course, this is by no means the first book on the subject. There are important texts about the addictions on which I have relied for information and critical comment. Being an addictions enthusiast, I belong to a number of fan clubs. My favourite stars are Nick Heather, Jim Orford, John B. Davies, Bill Miller, and Alan Marlatt. (There is a minor luminary called Harold Rosenberg, but I mention him only because he teaches at Bowling Green State University in the USA, and I expect him to recommend this book to his students.)

I benefited also from the help of colleagues and friends, who kindly read drafts of the manuscript and gave me invaluable advice. I am indebted to Professor Ray Cochrane, Series Editor, for reading the entire manuscript and providing helpful comments and encouragement to keep going. My friends and colleagues in the Psychology Department at Rampton Hospital were also keen advisers and supporters. Ray St Ledger deserves my thanks, and possibly even some tangible reward, for the considerable amount of time he spent reading drafts and giving advice. He was more generous still in supporting me when I got frazzled trying to write a book while also trying to keep abreast of my other work in the hospital. Mark Gresswell gave me the benefit of his extensive theoretical knowledge (self-reported), not to mention taunts about the book as a whole, which he retitled *All I Know About Addiction by Mary McMurran*. John Hodge disagreed with me, as usual, about dependence; I do not like to admit it, but I have learned a considerable amount from him during our debates on the subject. Finally, Mike Coogan, an organic chemist, provided a different perspective altogether. His trenchant comments and sound advice were extremely helpful to me, and he will be long remembered for his query 'Is talking bollocks in pubs a symptom of alcoholism?'

Mary McMurran
January 1994

References

HANKINSON, J. (1985) *Bluff Your Way in Philosophy*, Horsham, West Sussex, Ravette Books.

MURPHY, E.F. (1979) *The Macmillan Treasury of Relevant Quotations*, London, The Macmillan Press Ltd.

Chapter 1

Addiction:
Misconduct and Disease

Addiction is a term used in everyday language, usually without much reflection upon precisely what the construct means. Addressing the question 'What is addiction?' opens a Pandora's box of troublesome concepts which take some effort to define and understand. Informally, addiction may be defined as a degree of involvement in a behaviour that can function both to produce pleasure and to provide relief from discomfort, to the point where the costs appear to outweigh the benefits. Heavy involvement in an addictive behaviour is often accompanied by the recognition on the part of the 'addict' of the physical, social or psychological harm that he or she incurs, and an expressed desire to reduce or cease the addictive behaviour, yet, despite this, change is no easy matter.

The aim in this book is to explore the meaning of addiction to understand why some people continue to engage in a behaviour to the degree where the costs apparently exceed the benefits. As a first step in understanding what addiction is, we need to look at the historical development of the construct of addiction. Tracing the history of addiction shows that definitions of and responses to overindulgence have changed over time, depending not only on scientific knowledge but also on public attitudes and beliefs prevalent in any given place at a particular time.

Two important approaches to understanding behaviour, including addictions, have prevailed at different periods of time: the moral model and the disease model. The *moral model* of human behaviour is based on the notion of free will; people are presumed to be able to choose what they will do in a variety of situations. Behaviour which contravenes social norms is, therefore, seen as sinful, weak-willed, or simply a social nuisance (and perhaps a combination of all three). Based on the moral model, logical responses to undesirable behaviour are religious counselling, legislative controls and punishment. The moral model of behaviour prevailed in Britain and the United States in the eighteenth century, and the term addiction was at that time used simply to mean a bad habit or vice.

The *disease model* or *medical model* of human behaviour became prominent in the nineteenth century, the conditions for this change being created by developments in the natural sciences. Physicians borrowed the concepts employed in the new physics and chemistry and applied them to human behaviour. The notion of free will gave way to determinism; that is, every event, including human thoughts and actions, must have a cause, and we must look to science to provide information about the factors that determine that event. The most significant development was the application of medical concepts to problems that had previously been regarded as within moral or spiritual domains. Thus undesirable behaviours came to be viewed as the symptoms of physical malfunctions and, where no physical cause was apparent, the notion of 'mental illness' was evoked. When undesirable behaviour is thus construed as a disease, treatment rather than punishment is indicated.

The use of drugs was one type of behaviour which lent itself well to reconstruction from a moral failing into a disease: the disease called addiction. The disease model was seen as especially fitting to the explanation of behaviours that involved taking into the body substances that could be presumed to interfere with the body's natural chemistry. However the transition from the moral to the medical model was neither abrupt nor complete. Approaches to dealing with undesirable behaviour even today contain both moral and medical elements: legislation, punishment and religious exhortation coexist with medical interventions. In tracing the development of the construct of addiction, it is instructive to examine how the moral and medical models have applied differentially over time. It would be simple to launch straight into the history of responses to drug use, but first there is an important question to be asked: What is a drug?

What is a Drug?

Many substances, from aspirin to heroin, are classified as drugs; only some of these substances are called 'addictive' drugs. There is, in fact, no intrinsic characteristic that distinguishes drugs from non-drugs. We cannot look to chemistry to help us define a drug – there is no uniting chemical feature. Nor can we look to pharmacology for an answer in terms of effects on the human body – substances classified as drugs variously stimulate, sedate, cause hallucinations, alleviate pain, prevent infection, or anaesthetize. The concept of a drug is, in fact, a social artefact (Gossop, 1982). How a substance comes to be classified as a drug is a fascinating topic, the essence of which seems to be the determination of powerful social groups to control the use of particular substances for a variety of reasons. From some angles, it is clear that control over the use of some substances is imposed out of concern for the individual's physical well-being. From a different aspect, it is apparent that control over the use of certain substances is imposed because using them makes people troublesome. From yet another perspective, it may seem that controls are designed to aid the manufacture and distribution of substances that contribute to a nation's economy, and eliminate competition. Looking at the issue a different way, it may be that certain professional groups – doctors and pharmacists – wish to enhance their status and security in the world by keeping to themselves the powers of prescription and sale of specific substances.

The types of control exercised reflect one or more of these aspects of the need to control, thus we have legislation controlling possession, use and sale of drugs; taxation; mandatory public health warnings; and codes of practice for advertising. Where the control of substances called drugs is operating effectively, we tend to see those substances as good, or at least good if used appropriately or sensibly. Thus, tranquillizers are good drugs as long as a doctor prescribes them appropriately, and alcohol is beneficial as long as drinkers do not overindulge. Where controls are not operating effectively, the drugs concerned are labelled bad, for example with heroin, crack and ecstasy.

Szasz (1974) suggests that to call a drug 'addictive' is erroneously based on the notion that addiction is a condition caused by the chemical properties of the drug; he thinks that we call drugs 'addictive' because we see that people like to use them, particularly where the people involved belong to groups that readily lend themselves to social stigmatization. People seem to like to use the species of drug known as 'psychoactive drugs', that is 'any chemical substance, whether of natural or synthetic origin, which can be used to alter perception, mood, or other psychological states' (Gossop, 1982, p. 2). Davies (1992) notes that it is beyond doubt that certain substances have psychoactive effects, but that the notion of 'having to have' a drug cannot be explained by its pharmacology. He goes on to point out that, in the final analysis, there must be a physiological basis for *all* action, so the notion of 'having to have' a psychoactive drug simply on the basis of its effects on the body's physiological processes does not distinguish drug use from any other behaviour. Indeed, we shall see later on that non-substance-based behaviours, such as gambling and sex, have recently been admitted to the addictions field of study as a consequence of reducing the emphasis on the biological element of addiction.

Szasz (1974) defines drug abuse simply as 'socially disapproved pharmacological behaviour' (p. 9) and he goes on to say that the study of *drugs* is quite rightly within the domains of chemistry, pharmacology and medicine, however the study of *drug use and drug avoidance* – what Szasz calls 'ceremonial chemistry' – does not fit within these domains. He illustrates his point well when he suggests that pharmacology is to drug use as gynaecology is to sex, or as mathematics is to gambling.

Primed with this knowledge that the classification of certain substances as drugs is a social convention, and not a natural, inviolable truth, and that the basis for addiction is not readily located within the pharmacology of any substance, let us turn now to the history of responses to drug use.

Bad Habits and Vices

If we look back at life in eighteenth-century Britain, the situation in relation to drug use was obviously quite different from that which pertains today. Alcohol was consumed in enormous quantities, and opium could be found on sale at the corner shop and was widely used as an analgesic.

In the eighteenth century, alcohol was seen as a good thing, but drunkenness and social disorder were not. Amongst the less elevated members of society, beer and gin were the common tipple. English brewers had learned to distil gin in the late seventeenth century and the populace took to the spirit with gusto, leading to what became known as the 'gin epidemic', which peaked around 1750. Much of the poverty and lawlessness amongst the working classes was blamed on excessive alcohol consumption. Taverns and gin palaces were meeting places for criminals and prostitutes, and habitual drunkenness became associated with crime, vice and public disorder (Shaw, 1982). Drunkenness was seen as a social problem and efforts were made to control the distillation and retail sale of gin through taxation and licensing (the Gin Acts of 1736 and 1743). Drunkards were controlled by punishment, including fines, whippings, stocks and imprisonment (Heather and Robertson, 1985).

In the same era – the eighteenth century – opium use in Britain was widespread and the drug was readily available from chemists, druggists, pharmacists, village shops, grocers, general stores and corner shops, usually in the form of laudanum – a mixture of opium and alcohol – but also in its raw form (Berridge, 1977). East Anglia in particular was noted to be an area of prodigious opium consumption, the main consumers being agricultural labourers and not the educated classes. In this damp, poorly drained region, neuralgia, rheumatism and the ague were commonplace and opium was the source of physical comfort (Orford, 1985). Opium use was readily tolerated because the drug was a panacea for the relief of many chronic ailments. Because people who used opium were not troublesome, as were many alcohol users, there was relatively little concern about the habit.

Industrialization

It is clear that in the eighteenth century, drug use was viewed as a social problem, if it was seen as a problem at all. Using opium was seen as a harmless means of managing ailments for which there existed no cure. Drinking alcohol, even in large quantities, was acceptable as long as the drinker did not get drunk and make a nuisance of himself or herself. But attitudes to drug use changed and to explain this we should acknowledge wider social changes occurring around this time.

The beginnings of the medicalization of alcohol and drug use must be seen against the background of the increasing industrialization of society. Prior to this, when the workforce was largely engaged in agricultural labour, the effects of drinking and drug use could be tolerated, but with the transition to industrial labour, drink and drugs were seen to interfere with work performance and safety. Progressive urbanization of the work force also increased the need for social control. Kohn (1987, p. 53) suggests that the affluent classes were

corralling the poor masses, organising them into streets, mills and factories. Yet inside those alleys and workshops, a class was taking shape which its masters could not understand. Its way of life, its conditions of existence, and above all its morals were therefore objects of fervid investigation.

In the early days of the Industrial Revolution when foundries, factories and mills were rapidly increasing in number, the typical employer was intent on accumulating capital to plough back into his business so that it could expand and develop; he did not spend his money on sumptuous living (Cole and Postgate, 1971). Because he made a virtue of moderation, he regarded it as a desirable characteristic in his employees. All of these issues – control, curiosity and middle-class values – combined in the expression of concern for the health and welfare of the working classes. The time was right for the advent of temperance.

Temperance

In the colonial US, the situation with regard to drink had been much the same as in Britain. Drink flowed freely and was considered the 'Good Creature of God'; drunkenness, however, was considered a sin. As industrialization progressed, the problems connected with alcohol use became more obtrusive, and the Quakers transformed the 'Good Creature' into the 'Demon Rum' (Keller, 1976). The hazards of alcohol became the focus of the temperance movement, whose proponents emphasized moderation for the greater good of society. A feel for the nature of temperance can be gained from the old joke about the temperance preacher who, in his lecture to the crowd, dropped a worm into a glass of whisky to illustrate the dangers of alcohol. The worm died and the preacher turned to the crowd and posed the rhetorical question, 'What does this tell you?' From the back of the hall, a cockeyed optimist responded, 'If you've got worms, drink whisky.'

The American Temperance Society was formed in 1826. The message of temperance spread to England, carried by seafarers to the port of Liverpool, where the Liverpool Temperance Society was formed in 1830. However, temperance had already been brought to Scotland by a Greenock magistrate, John Dunlop, who had visited France and been impressed by the moderation of the working classes there (Longmate, 1968). Dunlop founded a moderation society in 1828 or 1829, which spawned many branches throughout the west coast of Scotland. The foremost English crusader, however, was Joseph Livesey, a cheese merchant of Preston, who was the founder of the British Teetotal Temperance Society.

In Britain, temperance fitted well with the aim of educating the working classes, embodied in the Society for the Diffusion of Useful Knowledge. The creed of this society was that ignorance, idleness and debauchery were the enemies of the working man and that his asset – his labour – could be improved in value through education, hard work and temperance. Until its demise in 1847, the society published books and pamphlets on a variety of subjects, a tradition continued in the 1850s and 1860s by Trades Union publications, with the typical message to 'get intelligence instead of alcohol – it is sweeter and more lasting' (Cole and Postgate, 1971).

In the USA, the temperance movement, in alliance with Protestant religions, gained political momentum and it became a prohibition movement. The Reverend Howard Hyde Russell was one person responsible for changing the emphasis of the movement towards prohibition, by identifying the saloon as the centre of drunkenness, vice and corruption (Paredes, 1976). Soon, all alcohol use came to be seen as dangerous and no one was exempt from its damaging effects. A Prohibition Party emerged, whose manifesto was the total ban on the manufacture, sale, transportation and importation of alcoholic beverages. In 1919, success was achieved with the Eighteenth Amendment to the US Constitution that made these acts crimes. Prohibition was successful in reducing alcohol consumption and alcohol-related problems, yet it was an unpopular law since prohibition was difficult to enforce and gave rise to nationwide gangsterism that we associate with the USA of the 1920s. Public opinion against enforced abstinence swelled and Prohibition was repealed in 1933.

Where opium use was concerned, the man who precipitated public concern in Britain was Thomas De Quincey (1785–1859) who began publishing his essays *The Confessions of an English Opium Eater* in 1821 in the *London Magazine*. In the preface to his collected edition of *The Confessions* (reproduced in the 1907 edition), De Quincey extolled opium as 'the one sole *catholic* anodyne which has hitherto been revealed to man' and he also considered it to be a powerful counteragent to 'the formidable curse of *taedium vitae*' (p. 5). As an opium eater, he was in the prestigious company of the Romantic poets of that age – Coleridge, Byron, Keats and Shelley. However, De Quincey's writings gave rise to some concern about opiate use among the working classes, particularly for recreational rather than medicinal purposes (Berridge, 1979). He

7

commented, for example, on Manchester cotton workers who crowded druggists' shops on Saturday evenings to buy opium because their low wages would not stretch to the purchase of ales or spirits. De Quincey thought that wage increases would not change matters: 'I do not readily believe that any man, having once tasted the divine luxuries of opium, will afterwards descend to the gross and mortal enjoyments of alcohol' (p. 5).

Medical interest in opium use was fuelled by the death of the Earl of Mar in 1828 (Berridge, 1979). The Earl died of jaundice and dropsy two years after taking out a life-insurance policy. The insurance company at first refused to pay out on the grounds that the Earl was a regular opium eater and that this habit would have shortened his life. This case, along with the high number of infant deaths attributed to the practice of sedating babies with opium, led to investigations into opium use by the medical profession. This eventually resulted in the 1868 Pharmacy Act, which placed restrictions on prescription and sale of opium. Berridge (1977) places this legislation in context when she points out that public health considerations were only part of the force leading to the control of opium; the increase in the organization of professional groups at this time meant that physicians wanted to control prescribing and pharmacists wanted to control sales.

While opium eating and drinking were arousing concern about public health, a different type of opprobrium was directed toward another form of opium use: opium smoking. In both Britain and the US, immigrant Chinese were seen as proprietors of sinister opium dens where vice and debauchery were rife. This may have been an overdramatic view. It has been suggested that smoking opium was simply part of the Chinese way of life and to call the venues where smoking opium occurred 'opium dens' would be akin these days to calling places where people smoke cigarettes 'tobacco dens' (Kohn, 1987). Nevertheless, the anti-opium smoking attitude was common in England where the Chinese population amounted to a few hundred; in the US, there were thousands of Chinese immigrants and the fear of 'drug fiends' was intense (Kohn, 1987). Szasz (1974, p. 76) suggests that the Chinese immigrants were 'exceptionally hard-working and law-abiding people' and therefore their peculiar habit of opium smoking became the focus of the persecution simply because 'Americans could not admit that they hated and feared the Chinese because the Chinese worked harder and were willing to work for lower wages than they did.' Animosity toward opium smoking, undoubtedly with its roots in racism, may be seen as the origin of social ostracism of the 'drug addict'.

Disease of the Will

As has been shown, public concern about alcohol and drug use originated variously from needs to control the work force, stamp out lawlessness and keep immigrants in their place. It is also true that concern for the health of the population was important and members of the medical profession were therefore engaged in the study of alcohol and drug use. Trained in the management of disease as they were, it is hardly surprising that they looked at drug use and the problems associated with it from the medical perspective. It is worth emphasizing here that the disease model of addiction is one in which the behaviour itself is seen as a disease symptom; that is drinking and drug use are seen as symptoms of alcoholism or drug addiction. Davies (1992) points out the fundamental error in construing purposeful behaviours in disease terms when he highlights the difference between disease symptoms like high temperature, breathlessness or a rash, which are involuntary, and the 'symptoms' of going into a pub and buying a pint of beer, or sticking a needle into your arm, which are voluntary. To hit his point home, he asks, 'Is it reasonable to conceive of the practice of injecting insulin as a symptom of diabetes?' (p. 48).

Szasz (1974) suggests that the medical profession may well have started by treating 'disagreeable conduct and forbidden desire' *as if* they were diseases, that is using disease as a *metaphor.* However, over time, the metaphor became literal and the medical profession came to insist that 'disapproved behaviour was not merely *like* a disease, but that it *was* a disease – thus confusing others, and perhaps themselves as well, regarding the differences between bodily and behavioral "abnormalities" ' (Szasz, 1974, p. 5). Looking at the disease model of addiction in this way, it can be seen how construing the behaviours as a disease differs from the concern about the problems which those behaviours cause. Where drug use is concerned, there *are* health implications, and the medical profession is rightly involved in the matter. Davies (1992), who has a way with words that illustrates exactly the points he wishes to convey, says 'For example, during the late nineteenth and early twentieth centuries, missionaries went to Africa where many of them caught malaria and died. The disease was malaria; not the decision to go to Africa' (p. 48).

It is time now to turn to medical responses to alcohol and drug use. The first construction of excessive drinking as a disease was postulated by Benjamin Rush (1745–1813) a physician of Philadelphia in the US. In a paper first published in 1785, called *An Inquiry into the Effects of Ardent Spirits upon the Human Body and Mind*, he described addiction to spirits (not beer or wine) as a 'disease of the will'. Rush saw alcohol as the causal agent in the development of addiction, and he believed that drinking spirits could produce a craving over which the drinker was powerless, leading to loss of control over consumption and he prescribed total abstinence as the only cure for habitual drunkenness. His suggested methods of persuading drunkards to abstain from alcohol included plunging the body into cold water, severe whippings and shaming. Rush's theories were taken up by the American temperance movement in support of their cause.

Excessive drinking was also receiving attention from the medical profession in Europe. Thomas Trotter (1760–1832), an Edinburgh physician, published his doctoral dissertation in 1804, entitled *An Essay, Medical, Philosophical, and Chemical, on Drunkenness*. His views, although similar to those of Rush in the US, are seen as having been formulated independently. Trotter considered habitual drunkenness to be a 'disease of the mind' and recommended total abstinence from all alcohol, not just spirits. In Germany in 1819, Bruhl-Cramer coined the term 'dipsomania'. In 1838, the French psychiatrist, Esquirol, classified habitual drunkenness as a 'monomania'. In 1852, Magnus Huss, a Swedish professor of medicine, provided the world with the term 'alcoholism'.

It was not until the second half of the nineteenth century that the disease theory of addiction to drugs other than alcohol gathered strength. Morphine, the active ingredient of opium, had been isolated in 1803 but it was the advent of the hypodermic method of morphine administration in the 1850s that is seen as the important factor in the emergence of the concept of addiction. It was soon noticed that injections of morphine created an 'artificial want' and the condition of 'morphinism' was identified, with 'morphinists' being particularly prevalent amongst doctors themselves (Berridge, 1979). Eduard Levinstein, a German physician, is generally credited with the first formulation of the disease model of drug addiction with his publication of *Die Morphiumsucht* in 1877, which was translated and published in English the following year entitled *Morbid Craving for Morphia*. In this book, Levinstein was not simply issuing a warning about the side effects of the medication; he was describing a *disease* of morphinism (Parssinen, 1983). Levinstein's cure for the morphia habit bore some resemblance to Rush's cure for alcohol addiction in its severity; his advice was abrupt and immediate withdrawal effected by locking drug users in a room guarded by male warder-nurses. This treatment was enthusiastically adopted by English physicians, so much so that it became known as the 'English treatment' (Berridge, 1979).

Inebriety

Those movements against alcohol and drug use that emerged during the first part of the nineteenth century were able to gain strength for their arguments by drawing upon medical opinion. Temperance and prohibition, essentially moralistic movements, gather into their arguments the medical profession's theories about addiction as a disease to add weight to their influence. We can see that in doing this moral views about drinking and drug use became enmeshed with the medical perspective. Hitherto, addiction to alcohol and addiction to other drugs had, by and large, been separate areas of study. The disease models of drinking and drug use became linked with each other in the concept of inebriety.

The Society for the Study of Inebriety was formed in Britain in 1884, and its president was physician Norman Kerr (Berridge, 1979). After duly studying inebriety, Kerr formulated his theory; inebriety was, he concluded, a disease of the nervous system, allied to insanity, characterized by an irresistible impulse to indulge in intoxicating liquors or other narcotics. The disease took different forms according to the substance used – there was alcoholomania, opiomania, morphinomania, and so on. The significant point about Kerr's work, according to Berridge (1979), is that he succeeded in uniting the diseases of alcohol addiction and drug addiction both with each other and with mental illness. The disease of addiction was therefore free to enter the domain of the psychiatrist.

An interesting irony, given the aforementioned scorn British people poured upon its immigrant Chinese opium smokers, is that Britain at this time was the main opium supplier to China itself. Opium was grown in India and the British East India Company was the trade link with China, with the British economy relying heavily on the income from opium. Imports of opium into China had been banned since 1729, except under licence for medical use, and the East India Company plied its trade on the black market by selling opium to smugglers who ran their illicit cargo to China. The Chinese authorities resented the persistence of the British in flouting their law and the quarrel escalated into the Opium War of 1840–42. In Britain, there was a move against involvement in opium trading with China, leading to the formation in 1874 of the Society for Suppression of the Opium Trade. While the main purpose of this society was to fight against Britain's Indo-Chinese connection, its moral arguments nevertheless influenced English attitudes to addiction. The society counted amongst its membership many leading medical men who, in speaking on the society's behalf, emphasized the disease model of drug addiction, based on Kerr's theories.

Berridge (1979) points out that around this time the disease theory of addiction was a hybrid; addiction was both a disease *and* a vice.

> The continuing moral component ensured a disease theory which was individually oriented, where the addict was responsible, through volition, for his own condition. Addiction was 'medicalised', but failure to achieve a cure was a failure of self control, not medical science. (Berridge, 1979, p. 77)

The disease theory of addiction was to change considerably, however, and to understand the change we must look first to the study of alcoholism in the US after the repeal of Prohibition.

Classic Disease Model of Alcoholism

Prohibition in the US was repealed in 1933, in response to a ground swell of public antipathy. With alcohol once again freely available in the US, problems relating to drinking and drunkenness began to emerge. A new approach to these problems was needed since the public would not have tolerated any further legislative control and so the time was ripe for a resurgence of the disease model of alcoholism.

In 1935, Alcoholics Anonymous (AA) was formed by two men struggling to maintain their own sobriety. Bill W., a stockbroker, was a man whose career had suffered as a consequence of his heavy drinking. On one of his frequent visits to hospital to dry out, he experienced a spiritual revelation; he realized that he would only achieve sobriety by admitting to himself and God that he was powerless over alcohol. During his first months of sobriety, he noticed that he felt less tempted to drink when he was helping other drinkers by passing on his message of enlightenment to them. Later, Bill W. made a trip to Akron, Ohio, where yet another of his business ventures met with failure. He was tempted to drown his sorrows in alcohol, but made a last-ditch effort to maintain his sobriety by contacting a local church, asking to be put in contact with another alcoholic. He was introduced to a local physician, Dr Bob, and together they supported each other and formed the self-help fellowship that we know now as AA.

The AA ideology was based on a mixture of ideas, described by Fingarette (1989) as pseudomedical, psychological and religious, the most significant proposition being that 'alcoholics' are a specific group of people with an inherent vulnerability to alcohol. According to AA teaching, most people can drink moderately without any problem, but there are some people who have a biological vulnerability to alcohol, rather like an allergy, where even one drink causes them to crave alcohol and lose control over their drinking. Alcoholism is a disease which is progressive, irreversible and incurable. Although there is no cure for this loss of control over drinking, fortunately the condition may be arrested through abstinence. There are three significant points about this new approach: first, the cause of the disease is located firmly *within the individual,* and thus the general hazards of the agent, alcohol, and the influence of the environment are minimized; second, alcohol is seen to precipitate the phenomenon of *craving* with consequent *loss of control* over drinking, so that the alcoholic is compelled to drink regardless of the consequences; and third, the disease is assumed to be *irreversible* and so abstinence is the only possible, and necessarily lifelong, therapeutic goal.

During Prohibition, the medical profession had lost interest in the study of drunkenness, but after repeal when alcohol-related problems once more became evident the interest of the medical profession was rekindled. Jellinek, a physiologist, was invited to Yale University in the late 1930s to lead research in this area. There are two interesting guiding factors relevant to early research by Jellinek's group. First, the disease model of alcoholism was deliberately adopted as a strategy to avoid the social stigma attached to excessive drinking; this helped to attract both 'alcoholics' into treatment and funds for setting up the treatment service. Second, the research was conducted in close liaison with AA members, that is with a select subgroup of people who had experienced alcohol-related problems and who understood those problems to be related to a disease process. It is hardly surprising then that, at least in his early research, Jellinek arrived at a disease model of alcoholism that was remarkably similar to that of AA. It must be said that Jellinek was neither naive nor fraudulent – he stated that the disease model was an hypothesis and that his data were limited – however, his work was interpreted by others with considerably less caution.

Jellinek (1952) differentiated between 'alcohol addicts' and 'excessive drinkers'; only the addicts experience loss of control over drinking and it is here that the disease model applies. Jellinek reserved judgment about whether there was an innate predisposing factor that could explain loss of control, or if this was acquired as a result of excessive drinking. Heather and Robertson (1981, p. 8) summarize Jellinek's description of the emergence of alcohol problems as 'a series of barriers which less serious types of problem drinkers successively fail to surmount, leaving only the alcohol addict at the finishing line.' In Jellinek's terms, there is a continuum from a prealcoholic phase (relief drinking), through a prodromal phase (preoccupation with alcohol), to the crucial phase (loss of control over drinking), and finally to the chronic phase (incapacitation).

Jellinek then began to work extensively for the World Health Organization (WHO) and had the opportunity of studying drinking in greater depth and in various cultures across the world. His model of alcoholism, therefore, developed over the years to his influential book of 1960, *The Disease Concept of Alcoholism*. Here he acknowledged that drinking habits varied widely and he therefore defined 'alcoholism' as 'any use of alcoholic beverages that causes any damage to the individual or society or both'. He described five types of alcoholism, which he labelled with letters of the Greek alphabet:

- *alpha alcoholism* is drinking to relieve physical or mental pain, which creates social or psychological problems, but where no withdrawal symptoms are evident;
- *beta alcoholism* is regular heavy drinking, often in accordance with cultural norms, causing physical damage;
- *gamma alcoholism* is where the alcohol has caused biological changes, such as altered metabolism, leading to withdrawal symptoms, craving and loss of control over drinking – once the gamma alcoholic starts drinking, he or she cannot stop;
- *delta alcoholism* is like gamma alcoholism in respect of biological changes, but here the withdrawal symptoms are such that alcohol is always necessary – the delta alcoholic drinks constantly; and
- *epsilon alcoholism*, which is binge drinking, with drinking bouts separated by periods of abstinence.

Only gamma and delta alcoholism were considered to be disease forms, that is only they entailed biological changes (adaptation of cell metabolism, increased tissue tolerance and withdrawal symptoms) whose consequences were craving and loss of control or inability to abstain. The other forms of alcoholism, although problematic, were not disease forms. Thus, both in the AA ideology and in Jellinek's work we see the distinction drawn between alcoholics, who are supposedly in the grips of a disease process, and alcohol abusers, who may be causing harm to themselves or others but are not afflicted with the disease, a dichotomy that is central to later psychiatric classification systems.

Addiction to Drugs Other Than Alcohol

Two developments that significantly contributed to the development of the disease model in relation to drugs other than alcohol were the manufacture of a synthetic opiate named heroin and the isolation of cocaine from the coca plant. Heroin was marketed in 1898 by Bayer Pharmaceuticals as a medication for respiratory ailments. This new cough medicine was thought to possess all the therapeutic benefits of morphine, without the habit-forming dangers. Indeed, heroin was then used in the treatment of morphinism in the way that methadone (another synthetic opiate) is used today in the treatment of addiction to heroin. Cocaine was isolated in 1844 and used as a general tonic, treatment for sinusitis and hay fever, and as a cure for the opium, morphine and alcohol habits (Musto, 1973). This practice of treating habitual drug use by substituting one drug for another was to continue as new chemicals were manufactured. New drugs are usually promoted as less 'addictive' than whatever drug it is suggested they replace – a powerful marketing strategy on the part of pharmaceutical companies who, after all, stand to make considerable profits from drug sales.

In Britain, it was during the First World War that attention was paid to drug use, leading to a number of acts and committees which finally crystallized the disease model of addiction. In London, the recreational use of cocaine by soldiers on leave aroused fears for the war effort, particularly since the use of cocaine appeared to be linked with the use of the services offered by prostitutes. Controls over drugs were imposed by amendments to the Defence of the Realm Act (DORA, 1916), when it became an offence to supply drugs to any member of the armed forces. With the end of the war in 1918, DORA expired and its drug regulations became the basis of the Dangerous Drugs Act (1920) and the Dangerous Drugs Regulations (1921). These acts restricted possession of drugs and controlled doctors' prescribing practices.

Following the drug legislations, it became clear that some doctors were receiving large quantities of drugs that they were prescribing to patients, not to treat some organic disease, but to enable people who had become addicted to drugs to satisfy their craving (Spear, 1982). The Rolleston Committee, which was set up in 1924 to assist the Home Office in carrying out the law relating to drugs addressed itself to whether this was, in fact, proper medical treatment. The Rolleston Report of 1926 contained a statement which shaped British attitudes to addiction: 'the condition must be regarded as a manifestation of a disease, and not a mere form of vicious indulgence. In other words, the drug is taken not for the purpose of obtaining positive pleasure, but in order to relieve a morbid and overpowering craving' (cited by Kohn, 1987, p. 86). Maintenance prescription was, therefore, established as a medical treatment, to become known as the 'British system'.

Szasz's (1974) description of the position in the US reveals an altogether less liberal situation. The Harrison Act, passed in 1914, outlawed the sale of opium and its derivatives, which became available only through doctor's prescription for the treatment of disease. However, it came to the attention of the Federal Bureau of Narcotics and Dangerous Drugs that doctors were prescribing drugs to patients who complained of various ailments but without conducting physical examinations first. Szasz (1974, p. 150) states that 'In a series of Supreme Court decisions following the passage of the act, the Court declared that dispensing or prescribing opiates to addicts is outside the scope of legitimate medical practice and therefore also illegal.' Since maintenance prescription was illegal, heroin trading took place on the black market in the US.

Musto (1973) suggests that the Supreme Court decision to ban maintenance prescription led to the medical profession questioning whether or not addiction was a bona fide disease. Just as earlier doctors had drawn on new developments in the physical sciences for their paradigms, so did their 1920s counterparts draw on new developments; this time, they had psychoanalysis to look toward. Freud had shown how the subconscious had a strong hold on conscious behaviour, therefore the cause of addiction might be psychological – a functional neurosis. This view was supported by the apparent lack of power of medicine to cure addiction. A psychiatrist by the name of Lawrence Kolb, writing in 1923, suggested that there were two types of addict. There were those who had become addicted by accident through being introduced to drugs as a medication for an illness; such casualties of the system were reduced in number thanks to the Harrison Act. There were also those who were addicted by choice, which was not something that a normal person would choose to do; the addict by choice was a 'psychopath' and addiction was only one aspect of the condition, which also included criminal activity and social ineptness.

During that time when the classic disease model of alcoholism was being formulated in the 1950s and 1960s, the use of illicit drugs was again on the rise. Jazz, introduced to Britain from the US in the years just after the First World War, had gained a reputation for being popular with people who not only enjoyed the music, but also enjoyed taking heroin and indulging in sexual orgies; jazz was denounced by the church and the media as a corrupter of youth. During the Second World War, jazz clubs in London were seen as dens of vice and, like the opium dens of a century before, there was a racial element involved. Jazz was, of course, the music of black Americans, originating in the southern states, and amongst the American servicemen stationed in Britain during the war were black GIs. Jazz 'dives' were where blacks, whites and drugs met in an unholy combination.

The Home Office began to record the number of heroin addicts in 1954 and the numbers of registered addicts steadily increased over the years until in 1958 the Ministry of Health convened an Interdepartmental Committee on Drug Addiction – the Brain Committee – to update the Rolleston Report (Kohn, 1987). The first report of the Brain Committee (1961) strongly condemned maintenance prescription of heroin to addicts by doctors under conditions of inadequate medical supervision (Spear, 1982). Strong condemnation was, however, not sufficient to stop the practice. Some doctors were seen to be overprescribing and registered addicts were selling their surplus heroin on the black market, introducing people to the habit. The second report of the Brain Committee (1965) recommended that the legitimate supply of heroin should be drastically curtailed. Consequently, the Dangerous Drugs Act was amended in 1967 to restrict heroin prescription to doctors working at special drug treatment centres that opened in 1968 (Plant, 1987). The Brain Committee compared addiction to infectious diseases that must be declared to the authorities so that action may be taken to control their spread. The important issues, as the Committee saw them, were 'that the addict is a sick person and that addiction is a disease which (if allowed to spread unchecked) will become a menace to the community' (cited in Kohn, 1987, p. 102).

By this time, in addition to heroin and cocaine, a variety of other drugs had become more widely available, including amphetamines, cannabis, LSD (lysergic acid diethylamide) and barbiturates. Concern about drug use was widespread, yet in the 1960s and 1970s the disease model of addiction was steadily being challenged by newly emerging professional groups – the social scientists. In short, drinking and drug use were coming to be seen as under the influence of social and psychological factors as much as anything else, and so the search for an inherent disease factor was seen as futile. More attention will be given to the evidence from the social sciences later in the chapter, but it makes sense first to bring the history of the disease model up to date.

Substance Dependence

Again, it was the field of alcohol studies that led in conceptual development. Faced with the evidence that drinking had a range of causes and effects, the medical profession had either to accommodate this or relinquish the disease model of addiction. Of course, they accommodated. In the late 1970s, the World Health Organization (WHO) brought together a group of experts to address the growing difficulties inherent in the term alcoholism that did not take into account the broad spectrum of physical, psychological and social factors related to drinking (Shaw, 1982). Two members of the WHO team of experts, the English psychiatrist Griffith Edwards and his American colleague Milton M. Gross, collaborated to produce in 1976 a new formulation of what had been previously understood as 'alcoholism' – the alcohol dependence syndrome.

Edwards and Gross (1976) presented the alcohol dependence syndrome as a 'clinical impression' and, although they state that it is 'difficult to link the clinical syndrome with information on the psychobiological basis of dependence', they mention enigmatically that 'scientific understanding has advanced recently' (p. 1058). The syndrome is a cluster of seven elements that concur; not all the elements need to be present, nor present with the same intensity. The elements are:

1   *narrowing of the drinking repertoire*, that is the dependent person, unlike the non-dependent drinker, begins to drink to the same extent whether it is a work day, weekend or holiday, and irrespective of whether he or she is alone or in company, and whatever his or her mood;

2   *salience of drink-seeking behaviour*, that is the individual gives priority to drinking above other activities;

3   *increased tolerance to alcohol*, that is increasingly more alcohol is required to experience the same effect, although in later

stages of dependence this tolerance declines and the drinker becomes incapacitated by quantities of alcohol that he or she could previously hold easily;

4 *repeated withdrawal symptoms*, that is tremor, nausea, sweating and mood disturbance;

5 *relief or avoidance of withdrawal symptoms by further drinking*, that is drinking first thing in the morning to get going, or constantly remaining topped up with alcohol so that symptoms of withdrawal are never experienced;

6 *subjective awareness of compulsion to drink*, that is the knowledge that once a drink is taken, further drinks will follow, despite the awareness that this is irrational, and a compulsive rumination on alcohol when experiencing withdrawal; and

7 *reinstatement after abstinence*, that is, although abstinence may be possible, once drinking starts there is rapid return to previous levels of consumption.

Shaw (1979), in his critique of the alcohol dependence syndrome, pointed out some fundamental shortcomings of the concept. First, loss of control was retained as a key feature of the syndrome, despite evidence for this being equivocal. Second, although the syndrome suggests gradients of dependence, a cut-off point between dependent and non-dependent is taken to exist; that is, gradients of dependence apply only to those people already classified as dependent. Third, the concept of dependence diverts attention away from the complexities of why people drink heavily by concentrating upon internal factors and minimizing situational and interpersonal factors. Nevertheless, this concept of dependence was quickly adopted into psychiatric classification systems to define the core element of psychoactive substance use disorders – that is for *all* psychoactive drugs, not just alcohol. It is instructive to note that this widespread adoption of the dependence syndrome occurred in the absence of supporting empirical evidence. The syndrome is something of an article of faith.

Psychiatric Classifications

Before moving on to present some of the challenges to the disease model of addiction, a brief summary of the psychiatric classification of addiction will be given, since this virtually summarizes the history of the construct. There are two main systems of classification of psychiatric disorders: the American Psychiatric Association's (APA) *Diagnostic and Statistical Manual of the Mental Disorders* (DSM), and the World Health Organization's (WHO) *International Classification of Diseases* (ICD). Both systems are constantly being updated, and DSM is in its fourth incarnation (actually called DSM-III-Revised) while ICD is in its ninth.

Diagnostic and Statistical Manual of Mental Disorders (DSM)

Alcoholism and drug dependence appeared in DSM-I (APA, 1952) and DSM-II (APA, 1968) as subsets of the category 'sociopathic personality disturbance', along with antisocial behaviour and the sexual deviations (Nathan, 1991). This mixed category clearly shows how behaviours that may be a threat to good order in society have been pathologized; the moral and disease models meet. DSM-III (APA, 1980) was particularly important since there was a move away from the implicit moralizing by allocating a separate category to the substance use disorders, within which two types of disorder figure – abuse and dependence. Abuse was defined by impaired social or occupational functioning, whereas dependence was defined by the presence of tolerance and withdrawal. DSM-III shows clear links with Jellinek's model. In the revision of DSM-III, known as DSM-III-R (APA, 1987), the abuse and dependence types of disorder were retained, but dependence was redefined using Edwards and Gross's (1976) alcohol dependence syndrome as a basis and applied to all types of psychoactive substance, not just alcohol. Within the substance use disorders category various substances are mentioned specifically: alcohol, amphetamine, cannabis, cocaine, hallucinogens, inhalants (e.g. gas, glue, paint thinners), nicotine, opioids, phencyclidine (PCP), and sedative, hypnotic, or anxiolytic drugs (e.g. sleeping pills and tranquillizers).

International Classification of Diseases (ICD)

The ICD is a statistical classification not only of mental disorders but also of physical conditions, which was originally used in the classification of causes of death. It originated in 1893, with the first revision in 1900 and regular revisions at approximately ten year intervals thereafter.

Up until 1948, alcohol and drug-related problems were classified under 'Chronic poisoning and intoxication'. ICD-6 (WHO, 1948) contained the first separate section on mental disorders, developed for the classification of psychiatric casualties of World War II (Kramer, 1988). In ICD-6 and ICD-7 (WHO, 1955), alcoholism and drug addiction appeared in the category 'Disorders of character, behaviour, and intelligence'. As part of the preparatory work for ICD-8, WHO commissioned a study of the classification of the mental disorders in recognition of the fact that they represented a major international health problem. To this end, a number of expert committees were formed to discuss classification and nomenclature.

Alcoholism and drug dependence appeared in ICD-8 (WHO, 1965) within the category 'Neuroses, personality disorders, and other non-psychotic mental disorders'. In ICD-9 (WHO, 1977), within the same overall category, three separate disorders were listed: the alcohol dependence syndrome, drug dependence and nondependent abuse of drugs.

Challenges to the Disease Model

It is time now to look at challenges to the disease model of addiction; a summary of the main tenets of that model will guide our thinking here. Central to the disease model of addiction is the concept of *loss of control* over substance use; that is, a substance user may be observed to engage heavily and repetitively in drug-taking behaviours, and expresses a feeling of powerlessness over his or her drinking or drug use. The concept of loss of control is predicated upon three assumptions:

1   that repeated drug use leads to *tolerance* to that substance, that is there is a need to increase the dosage to gain the same effects;
2   that when the effects of the drug wear off, the user will experience *withdrawal symptoms*, such as tremor, hot flushes, nausea, cramps and delirium, which are alleviated by taking the drug; and

3 that hand in hand with physical withdrawal goes the psychological phenomenon of *craving*, that is a strong desire or compulsion to have the drug.

The disease model would suggest that addicts are different from the rest of us, having some biological or psychological abnormality that was either present in their constitution from the start or that has been triggered by use of the drug. This constitutional difference is irreversible, and the disease is progressive, therefore the only sensible course open to an addict is to abstain from the drug. Is the disease model a good way of describing drug-taking behaviour?

A model is simply a way of representing what is known about a subject, in this case alcohol and drug use. Clearly, any model must fit the observed data, that is it must represent accurately what may be observed about the subject it concerns. A model ought also to be useful in some way, that is it must allow for the generation of hypotheses that can be tested and thereby add to our knowledge of the subject. Where alcohol and drug use are concerned, a model will be useful if it allows for speculation relating to how alcohol and drug use develop over the course of time, how problems arise, and how we might intervene to prevent or alleviate problems. When these hypotheses are tested, they may be supported, in which case we would wish to retain that model, or they may be falsified, in which case we would reject that model and look for some other more useful way of integrating our knowledge. With relation to the disease model of addiction, some important observations and experimental findings raise doubts about its validity and utility. The main issues will be outlined below, without any pretence of being an exhaustive review of the relevant literature.

Is Addiction Irreversible?

The progressive nature of addiction postulated by the disease model is the tenet upon which abstinence is based; that is, once the disease gets a grip, there is no cure and the best one can do is arrest its progress through total abstinence. There is one glaring absurdity in this proposition: a person who is believed to have lost control of his or her substance use is expected to exercise sufficient control to abstain altogether. What is abstention if not control? This is not to deny that it may sometimes be easier to abstain completely than to maintain moderation, but simply to point out the strange logic of the disease model.

Where excessive drinking is concerned, there are now many studies that report normal drinking by people previously diagnosed as alcoholics and who have received abstinence-oriented treatment. In 1962, D.L. Davies reported a follow-up study of 93 'alcoholics' who had been in abstinence-oriented treatment at the Maudsley Hospital in London. Since their discharge from treatment – a period of between seven and 11 years – seven reported drinking in moderation without getting drunk or losing control. Despite the fact that the proportion of ex-patients who had gained control over their drinking was small, Davies's report led to an intense controversy. His critics suggested that this small group of controlled drinkers had been misclassified as alcoholics in the first place; that the recovered 'alcoholics' were not really drinking normally at all; that they were only on the road to a full-blown relapse; and that they were freaks in the sense of having a weird biochemistry, an unusual psychopathology, or a miracle cure (Heather and Robertson, 1981).

J.B. Davies (1992, p. 66) points out the absurdity of the argument that any recovered alcoholic was not an alcoholic in the first place when he says:

> Unfortunately, this implies that the known population of 'alcoholics' at any one time consists of two indistinguishable subgroups, 'real alcoholics' who are driven to drink by forces beyond their capacity to control and 'bogus alcoholics' who might decide to stop misusing alcohol at any moment.

Where the patient recovers, according to the circular logic of the argument, he/she never had 'it' in the first place and so these bogus 'alcoholics', says Davies, must have been drinking on purpose and at some point must have decided to stop.

A similar controversy was born in the USA out of what is known as the Rand Report. The government body called the National Institute on Alcohol Abuse and Alcoholism (NIAAA) had set up a number of Alcoholism Treatment Centers (ATCs) across the US, and a group of researchers at the Rand Corporation set out to conduct a four-year follow-up study of alcoholics treated in these ATCs. The subjects were 758 randomly selected males admitted to the ATCs in 1973. Four years later, data were collected on 85 per cent of the sample. In general, for those who were still alive (14.5 per cent had died), the data revealed that problem drinking was the most common pattern, occurring in 54 per cent of the sample. However, at the time, 46 per cent were in control of their drinking and had been for the past six months, 28 per cent through abstaining from alcohol and 18 per cent drinking variable amounts without any apparent problems as a consequence (Polich, 1980).

Closer investigation of individual patterns of drinking over the years revealed that instability was common; that is, both abstainers and non-problem drinkers would show periods of remission from drinking problems but would relapse again into problem drinking. It was this instability that impressed both the managers of the ATCs and the media at the time; the results of the Rand Report were taken to mean that 'alcoholics' cannot return to normal drinking. The assumption was that 'alcoholics' who were currently drinking without any problem were simply on the road to relapse, but the flaw in this conclusion is the implicit corollary that abstainers are *not* headed for a relapse. The actual findings presented in the Rand Report were that some 'alcoholics' managed to abstain for lengthy periods (7 per cent had abstained for the full four years of the study), but so did some 'alcoholics' manage to moderate their drinking for lengthy periods. The most common pattern however was one of repeated relapses into heavy drinking and this was true for those who attempted to abstain as well as for those who attempted to moderate their drinking (Armor, 1980).

An important observation in the study of addiction to opiates was afforded by the unfortunate circumstances of the Vietnam war. It was assumed that many American military personnel in Vietnam were using heroin, opium and other illicit drugs, and there was concern about the potential increase of the drug problem when they returned home. In 1971, mandatory urine screening was introduced for all soldiers returning to the US so that drug users could be identified and treated. Concern about the reintegration of drug users back into civilian life led to a follow-up study of Vietnam returnees.

Robins *et al.* (1975) interviewed a general sample of 470 returnees from Vietnam between eight and 12 months after their return. Before going to Vietnam, only 2 per cent had used heroin, yet during their stay almost half had taken some narcotic at least once and around 20 per cent were judged to have been addicted. After Vietnam, drug use decreased to preservice levels and only 7 per cent of users were identified as addicted. These 7 per cent experienced no problems in getting hold of drugs, and so lack of availability was ruled out as a reason for remission. Robins *et al.* (1975, p. 961) concluded that, with an addiction remission rate of 95 per cent, 'the opiates are not so addictive that use is necessarily followed by addiction nor that once addicted, an individual is necessarily addicted permanently.'

Observations that addiction was not irreversible led on to a closer investigation of the phenomena that were supposed to be the key features of the disease.

Conditioned Reactions

The first point to be made here is that tolerance and withdrawal are to some extent *situationally and psychologically determined*; that is these phenomena are not based exclusively on some predictable and fixed physiological mechanism. A number of interesting laboratory studies have been designed to investigate the relevant issues. Of course, because of legal constraints, alcohol has been the main drug used by researchers in human studies, whereas in the study of illicit drugs animals have been used as subjects.

While physiological changes do occur with repeated pharmacological stimulation, a complete account of drug tolerance and withdrawal requires an appreciation of environmental influences. For example, environmental specificity of tolerance to morphine has been examined in a series of experiments with rats (Siegel, 1988). First, tolerance to morphine was developed by giving the rats a series of morphine injections. In this tolerance development phase, administration of the drug was paired with consistent auditory and visual environmental cues. The rats were then divided into two groups for a tolerance test. After administration of a further dose of morphine, the degree of analgesia shown by the rat was measured, for example the time taken to lick its paw when placed on a hot plate (54 degrees Celsius), or the time taken to withdraw its paw from a source of increasing pressure. One group of rats received the tolerance test following the same audiovisual cues as were present during the tolerance development phase; the second group of rats received the tolerance test following different cues. In addition, a control group of rats, none of which had been administered any morphine and so had not developed tolerance, were given the tolerance test. Rats that were tolerance tested following the same cue conditions that signalled the drug during the tolerance development phase were *more* sensitive to pain than either of the other two groups of rats. That is, morphine tolerance is more pronounced under the environmental conditions associated with drug administration compared to an alternative environment.

Given alcohol Told alcohol	Given alcohol Told not alcohol
Not given alcohol Told alcohol	Not given alcohol Told not alcohol

Figure 1.1   *The balanced placebo design*

Experience of withdrawal symptoms in 'alcoholics' has been shown to occur upon exposure to physical alcohol cues, for example the sight and smell of drink (Pomerleau *et al.*, 1983). Where drug users are concerned, they report feeling cravings in response to pictures or videotapes of drug paraphernalia and drug injecting (Childress *et al.*, 1986). These studies indicate that tolerance and withdrawal may be conditioned reactions to environmental substance use cues; any distinctive environment that is repeatedly associated with a drug effect will eventually elicit a reaction.

This conditioning process also applies to internal cues, such as thoughts and emotions, as demonstrated in experimental studies. In 1966, Merry conducted an experiment that raised doubts about the physiological basis of craving. He gave 'alcoholics' an orange vitamin drink, in some cases laced undetectably with vodka and in some cases not, and then asked subjects to rate the strength of their craving for alcohol. He found no differences between those given alcohol and those not given alcohol. This suggests that craving is linked with the knowledge that alcohol has been consumed; that is, the drug ethanol does not trigger off some internal physiological mechanism that explains craving.

The cognitive element in loss of control has been clearly illustrated in experiments using what is known as the balanced placebo design. Here, subjects may be given alcohol with tonic water or just plain tonic water. Half of the subjects in each group are told they are drinking alcohol, and the other half are told they are drinking only tonic. This leads to four conditions, as shown in Figure 1.1, and enables researchers to separate out the belief that one has consumed alcohol from actual alcohol consumption. Marlatt *et al.* (1973), using the balanced placebo design, demonstrated that problem drinkers did not inevitably lose control over their drinking. Problem drinkers were given a drink along with instructions about the content of that drink. They were then invited to drink as much as they wished, supposedly to form an opinion about brand preference. Those who were told that they were drinking alcohol drank most, irrespective of whether their drinks actually contained alcohol or not. These findings suggest that it is the *belief* that alcohol is being consumed – not actual consumption – that triggers apparent loss of control.

Craving may be considered as a cognitive representation of withdrawal experiences (whether physiological or conditioned). Davies (1992) suggests that craving is just another word used to describe an experience of discomfort, and an accompanying desire to get rid of that discomfort. A craving explanation, says Davies (p. 51)

> is offered in circumstances where (i) people consistently choose to reduce their discomfort, and (ii) there is a consensus belief about the biological determinants of the discomfort. Thus, while drug users 'crave' (have to have) drugs and hungry people 'crave' food, people merely 'want' colour TV sets or holidays in Venice.

He suggests that it is this impression of an autonomous force whose power cannot be resisted that distracts from the reality that people either resist or indulge in drug-taking because they have good reasons for doing so.

Are There Differences between Addicts and Non-addicts?

One aspect of the search for a difference between addicts and non-addicts has been the quest to identify an 'addictive personality'. Nathan (1988) reviewed studies investigating three main kinds of link between personality and alcohol and drug abuse:

1 attempts to identify a personality type that precedes and therefore predicts substance abuse;
2 attempts to identify personality characteristics that are specific

to the disorder, that is differentiating substance abusers from non-abusers, or abusers of one kind of substance from another, or various levels of the problem; and

3   attempts to identify personality characteristics that predict treatment outcome.

His conclusions are that research findings have shown only one consistent finding: a correlation between antisocial behaviour in childhood and adolescence and 'alcoholism' in adulthood. He makes two points about this. First, it is antisocial *behaviour* not antisocial *personality* that has been identified as a precursor of 'alcoholism'. Second, high rates of antisocial behaviour in our society make this an inefficient predictor of 'alcoholism'; that is, given that large numbers of abusers have never demonstrated antisocial behaviour in childhood, and also that many antisocial children and adolescents do not go on to develop problems with alcohol in adulthood, the usefulness of antisocial behaviour as a predictor of 'alcoholism' is dubious. Many heavy users of drugs and alcohol also show signs of depression, which distinguishes them from people who do not abuse substances, but it seems that depression is a consequence of the drug use, relating either to the lifestyle or the pharmacological effects of the drug, rather than a central and lasting feature of the drug user. Nathan found no relationship between personality and response to treatment. Overall, his conclusions are that 'the utility of personality for the prediction of substance abuse, for the differentiation of substance abusers from non-abusers, and for determining the response to treatment and the maintenance of treatment gains remains unproven' (Nathan, 1988, p. 187).

Cook and Gurling (1990) have reviewed studies of genetic aspects of alcoholism and substance abuse. Owing to methodological problems of separating genetic from environmental factors, results are, at best, equivocal, and it is worth pointing out that no mechanism for genetic transmission has been identified. The strongest finding is that there is an increased likelihood of alcoholism in males adopted away from their alcoholic biological parents. Given the observed association between antisocial behaviour and alcoholism, and between depression and drug use in general, geneticists are speculating about a genetic predisposition to these personality disorders.

As Peele (1985) points out, the basic problem with genetic models of addiction is that they do not provide the answer to why people drink or take drugs. Even if a person is genetically programmed to overindulge, this does not prevent him or her experiencing the adverse effects of overindulgence. What stops him or her learning from experience?

An Alternative Model of Addiction

As we have just seen, there is sufficient evidence to suggest that the disease model of addiction does not fit the facts. Loss of control is not inevitable or invariable; tolerance, withdrawal and craving vary; 'addicts' are not different (except that they drink or use drugs excessively); and the problem is not necessarily irreversible or progressive. How, then, are we to understand addiction?

Biological theories, from which the medical model derives, and psychological theories of personality look *inside* a person to explain behaviour. A different approach is to explain behaviour in terms of the interaction between the person and the *outside* world. In doing so, psychologists see behaviour as *learned*. It is the purpose of the next chapter to give a detailed account of psychological models of addiction in order to set the scene for a thorough explanation of the psychology of addiction.

Chapter 2

Psychological Approaches to Addiction

Psychologists view behaviour – all kinds of behaviour and not just addictions – as determined by a multitude of factors. A list of factors that needs to be taken into account in explaining behaviour is presented Table 2.1. Our understanding of behaviour is not fixed upon any one factor, but acknowledges this range of influences operating simultaneously. Looking at this list, it should be quite obvious that the influences that determine behaviour will vary from one person to the next, and will vary for any one person over time. The influence of these broad factors can be readily illustrated in relation to substance use.

Table 2.1   *Factors that determine behaviour*

Culture
Family
Social group
Lifestyle
Environment
Behavioural skills
Thoughts
Feelings
Physical factors

Differences exist both between cultural groups and within any one cultural group across time in their laws and attitudes to drinking and drug use. We saw in the previous chapter how legislation to control alcohol and drug use developed over time in Britain and the US, and how alcohol was prohibited in the US between 1919 and 1933. Today, drinking alcohol is permitted in most western countries, yet it is prohibited in some countries, for example Saudi Arabia. We need look no further than the Netherlands for an example of a country today where the use of cannabis is not a criminal offence. A country's legal position in relation to substance use can influence an individual's consumption by affecting availability, restricting the opportunities for using a substance, and conveying cultural attitudes to substance use. Restrictions do not always take effect in the desired direction, however; for some people, the excitement and risk attached to illicit drug use may actually attract them toward this activity. Indeed, part of the reasoning behind the decriminalization of cannabis in the Netherlands was to make drug use boring, and this appears to have been achieved successfully since consumption there has declined since the 1970s (Nadelman, 1989). Various groups within society also arrange to convey messages about drinking and drug use, for example the annual 'Drinkwise' day and the 'Just Say No' campaign organized by health educators. The general point here is that cultural factors can influence a person's drinking and drug use in a number of ways.

Family and social factors also have an impact. People will vary in their drinking and drug use according to their upbringing and the company they keep. Messages about drinking and drug use are passed on from parents to children, rules are set about what is and what is not acceptable behaviour, and restrictions may be imposed regarding friendships. Drinking and drug use are not typically solitary activities (at least not in the early stages) and there is no doubt about peer influence relating to substance use.

It is obvious too that a person's lifestyle will have some impact upon substance use. Issues here include whether a person lives alone or with a partner, possibly with children, how much money is available to spend on drink and drugs, and how a person organizes his or her time in respect of work and leisure activities.

Environmental factors also have a role to play. There are differences in the likelihood of substance use depending upon where a person lives. In rural areas, drinking alcohol may require more effort than in cities because pubs, off-licenses, and supermarkets are far fewer and further between. Of course, the inclination to drink may be stronger in the country where, arguably, fewer opportunities exist for involvement in other activities. In certain urban areas illicit drugs may be easily obtainable and this constitutes a risk factor for illicit drug use. The person's situation too will exert an influence on behaviour; drinking and drug use will be affected by factors such as whether one is alone or in company, and the function of any gathering. For example, drinking alcohol is encouraged at a party, but discouraged at school.

Behavioural skills are also important. A person who is competent in various activities may have less need to drink or use drugs than a person without such competencies. Included here are social skills, work skills and leisure skills. The way a person thinks and feels may have a profound influence on drinking and drug use. This will include beliefs about the substance in question relating to how harmful it may be or how beneficial it may be, psychologically, socially and physically. The use of alcohol and drugs to manage moods and emotions is particularly important, for example in the reduction of tension and anxiety.

Finally, there are undoubtedly physical factors that bear an influence upon drinking and drug use. For example, there are genetically determined differences in alcohol metabolism. Low levels of the enzyme which breaks down acetaldehyde (the first metabolic product of alcohol) lead to a strong negative physical effect. As a consequence, people who experience this negative effect are biologically predisposed not to drink large quantities of alcohol. It seems, for instance, that Oriental races – the Chinese and Japanese – have a genetically-based metabolic sensitivity to alcohol; that is they respond quickly and intensely to alcohol, with a flushing response known as 'Oriental flushing' (Marshall, 1990). This metabolic characteristic seems to protect against heavy drinking. Another example is that women seem to be more susceptible to the effects of alcohol than men, perhaps because of metabolic and hormonal differences. Another good example is the chronic drinker who, through damage to the liver (the organ that breaks down alcohol) over a protracted period of heavy drinking, is no longer able to take alcohol in large amounts.

Somehow, this whole range of factors that influence behaviour must be taken into account in any approach to understanding addiction. Psychological theories help us understand the *processes* by which these factors bear influence. Any theory must, of course, fit the observable facts of the situation. Addictive behaviours are activities that vary both between people and within any one person across time; no one can become addicted without starting in the first place, but not everyone starts; not everyone who does start becomes addicted; and not everyone who becomes addicted stays addicted. Therefore, for any theoretical approach to fit the facts, it must describe the processes of initiation to, maintenance of, and dependence upon the use of any substance, and the processes involved in change.

A theoretical understanding of addiction is also of crucial importance in developing effective methods of intervention to control addictive behaviours and reduce associated problems. Without theory, the development of intervention techniques is based on nothing more than guesswork.

Now that we know the range of factors that must be accounted for in any psychological approach to explaining addictive behaviour, the relevant major psychological theories will be described. The theories summarized here all hold relevance for the addictive behaviours, but none is exclusive to them – they explain other behaviours equally well. It is important to note that there is no single all-encompassing theory of addiction; these theories must not be seen as mutually exclusive, but rather complementary to each other. Nor can any claim be made that these psychological theories explain everything about addictive behaviours; other fields of study, for example economics, sociology and physiology, have a contribution to make. Neither is any one theory the final statement on the subject; there is constant research and refinement in each field, as one would expect in any scientific arena.

Classical Conditioning

The principles of classical conditioning are based on the work of Ivan Pavlov (1849–1936). Pavlov was a physiologist studying the digestion of food in dogs, and part of his research was to measure how much dogs salivated when they were fed. He noticed that dogs in his experiments began to salivate as soon as they heard the clanking of the food pails. That is, they had learned to associate the arrival of the pail with food. This learning by association is now known as *classical conditioning*.

In his famous experiments with dogs, Pavlov showed that when food was given to a dog in association with the sound of a buzzer or a bell ringing, eventually the sound of the buzzer or bell alone would make the dog salivate. In classical conditioning terminology, the food is the *unconditioned stimulus* and the sound of the buzzer or bell is the *conditioned stimulus*. Salivation in response to food is the *unconditioned response*, and salivation to the sound of the buzzer or bell is the *conditioned response*.

The importance of conditioned responses in the addictions field are that specific stimuli, through being so often paired with substance use, may come to elicit a desire to indulge in substance use. Heather and Robertson (1981) provide an example of this. They describe the hypothetical case of an office worker who drinks after work and typically arrives home at around 9 p.m. By the time he gets home, the level of alcohol in his blood is beginning to drop, which leads to the desire for more alcohol to restore the pleasant feelings of intoxication. His response, therefore, is to go to the pub for another drink. Over time,

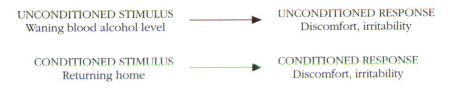

Figure 2.1 *The development of conditioned craving (After Heather and Robertson, 1981)*

returning home comes in itself to trigger the desire for alcohol. This process is described by Heather and Robertson in classical conditioning terms, as illustrated in Figure 2.1. The waning blood alcohol level (the unconditioned stimulus) leads to unpleasant feelings (the unconditioned response). These feelings occur at the time of returning home, and this becomes the conditioned stimulus, like the bell in Pavlov's experiment. By repeated association, returning home can in itself give rise to feelings of discomfort (the conditioned response) which are interpreted as a need for alcohol.

To return to the dogs for further elucidation, where the buzzer (the conditioned stimulus) is sounded over and over again, but food is no longer provided, salivation (the conditioned response) will diminish. This process is known as *extinction*. Procedures based upon extinction are used in the treatment of addictions, and are known as cue exposure with response prevention. What happens is that cues related to drinking or drug use are presented to the client, for example a glass of alcohol, injecting equipment or a substance that looks like a drug – powdered sugar or talc. No drinking or drug use is allowed to follow, with the aim of extinguishing the conditioned response of drug craving to the visual cues (conditioned stimuli). After extinction, the associations built up during conditioning are not completely forgotten and the phenomenon of *spontaneous recovery* can be observed. A good example here is the former smoker who may have extinguished the craving response after meals – the time when many smokers say they most enjoy a cigarette. Spontaneous recovery may occur after a particularly fine dinner under unusual circumstances, say during a summer holiday or at a celebration. The desire for a cigarette re-emerges and is indulged.

Responses to conditioned stimuli may *generalize*, that is a stimulus similar to the original unconditioned stimulus, but not identical to it, will elicit a response. However, there is evidence that organisms can also *discriminate* in that, if the stimulus becomes too different from the original unconditioned stimulus, then it will not elicit a response. A fascinating experiment by one of Pavlov's students illustrates generalization and discrimination. A dog was given food in association with a picture of a circle drawn on a card. The researcher noticed that the dog would salivate not only to the circle, but also to the picture of an ellipse (generalization). The researcher then went on to train the dog to discriminate between a circle and an ellipse by presenting food with the former and no food with the latter, finding that the dog did learn to salivate only to the circle (discrimination). A further stage was to present the dog with the circle in association with food, and a very wide ellipse, which was almost a circle, without food. The dog did discriminate between the two at first, but over time it was noticed that discrimination was not improving; in fact, it got worse until it finally disappeared altogether. The dog seemed to turn into a nervous wreck in that when it was taken into the laboratory it began to squeal, wriggle and destroy the apparatus with its teeth (Rachlin, 1970)!

Generalization and discrimination are important in addiction because feelings of craving conditioned to one particular set of circumstances may generalize to other situations. Looking back at Heather and Robertson's example of craving conditioned to arriving home at 9 p.m., this may generalize to coming home at any time, or being in the house at weekends. Clearly, training such a person to discriminate would be a useful intervention to restrict the circumstances under which drinking takes place.

Operant Conditioning

Operant conditioning models derive from the work of B.F. Skinner (1904–1990), whose research was devoted to understanding how behaviour operates upon the environment to produce changes that may be reinforcing or punishing. The term *operant* comes from the verb to operate. Behaviour is understood in terms of the consequences contingent upon it. That is, a behaviour is maintained – or not – as a result of its consequences. The study of the relationship between behaviour and its reinforcing or punishing consequences for any individual allows for these contingencies to be altered to reduce problem behaviour. This technique is known as contingency management.

Reinforcement is where the likelihood of a behaviour is increased; reinforcement may be positive, that is directly rewarding (e.g. physical satisfaction, providing material gain or leading to peer approval), or negative, that is avoiding or escaping aversive experiences (e.g. relief of physical, psychological or social discomfort). *Punishment* is where the likelihood of a behaviour is decreased; punishment may also be positive, that is directly aversive (e.g. physical pain, material loss or social disapproval), or negative, that is preventing the acquisition of positive outcomes (e.g. removing opportunities for physical, psychological or social satisfaction). Examples of these types of reinforcement and punishment in relation to drinking may help clarify the differences. Drinking may be *positively reinforced* by the 'buzz' a person gets from alcohol, and may be *negatively reinforced* by the relief of boredom. A hangover would be *positive punishment* and *negative punishment* would occur where a drinker who wishes to have sex is denied the pleasure through physical incapacitation.

Both reinforcement and punishment are defined by the relationship between a behaviour and its consequences. Where the behaviour is seen to increase, then the consequences are said to be reinforcing; where the behaviour is seen to decrease, then the consequences are said to be punishing. This is an important point which indicates that, in terms of operant conditioning, punishment does not necessarily relate to physical pain or suffering, although it can do in some cases. It is also important to note that there is individual variation in what is reinforcing and what is punishing. For example, the light-headed feeling that occurs after drinking is reinforcing for some people, but punishing for others. In most cases, there is a mixture of positive and negative outcomes, yet where a behaviour occurs we must take this as evidence that the positives outweigh the negatives.

In attempting to understand the power of reinforcement and punishment, it is important to take into account the frequency and regularity of the association. Taking the example of a cigarette smoker, each inhalation may be positively reinforced through stimulation of the pleasure centres in the brain, and negatively reinforced through elimination of the unpleasant feelings of nicotine deprivation. For a person smoking 20 cigarettes a day and taking 10 puffs per cigarette, reinforcement occurs 200 times per day. It is hardly surprising then that smoking becomes powerfully entrenched (Ashton and Stepney, 1982).

Another important aspect is the immediacy of the consequences. The reinforcement for smoking described above is happening within seconds of inhalation, and the close temporal association between smoking and satisfaction results in effective learning of that behaviour. By contrast, many of the negative consequences are not experienced until after a considerable delay in time; emphysema, bronchitis and lung cancer are not immediately consequent upon smoking.

As in classical conditioning, behaviour which ceases to be reinforced is extinguished. Differences in behaviour are also apparent in relation to patterns of reinforcement. One very important finding is that *partial reinforcement* produces greater resistance to extinction than continuous 100 per cent reinforcement. That is, if a behaviour is rewarded each and every time it occurs, when the rewards cease, extinction will be speedy. However, if a behaviour is rewarded only intermittently, that behaviour will persist through many unrewarded trials. Gamblers are often cited to illustrate this point. Playing a slot machine that paid out every time would be a boring, if remunerative, activity. No doubt the gambler would continue to feed the machine as long as it was paying out, but if it suddenly stopped paying out, then the gambler would soon pack up and go home. In real life, however, slot machines pay out intermittently and create excitement, if not wealth, for the gambler. In this case, if the machine were to stop paying out altogether, then the gambler would be likely to persist for a lot longer before going home.

Most behaviour does not occur at random; certain cues signal what the outcome is likely to be if a behaviour is carried out. These neutral stimuli in the environment are called *discriminative stimuli*. For example, there may usually be music playing in a particular pub where a person drinks regularly. Music could thus become a discriminative stimulus for drinking, since it signals that drinking will lead to having a good time. Generalization, a process already mentioned under classical conditioning, may occur where similar discriminative stimuli are encountered. In this case, any music may come to elicit drinking, for example drinking at home while listening to compact discs. Again, discrimination training would be helpful in reducing the behaviour in question.

Finally, the process of *chaining* is required to explain complex human behaviour. Complex behaviours consist of sequential component behaviours, where each component acts as both a cue (i.e. a discriminative stimulus) for the next behaviour in the chain, and a reinforcer (i.e. a conditioned reinforcer) for the preceding behaviour. For example, smoking a cigarette is a chain composed of buying a packet of cigarettes, taking a cigarette from the packet, lighting up, and inhaling the smoke. The primary reinforcer is the effect of nicotine upon the body. But taking a cigarette out of the pack and holding it in one's hand is also reinforcing for some people. Handling cigarettes is a conditioned reinforcer and also a cue for lighting up. Having a pack in one's pocket is a further link in the chain, as is buying cigarettes. Such chains are important in that the sooner they are interrupted, the easier it is to avoid the primary reinforcer. That is, it is probably easier not to buy a pack of cigarettes in the first place than it is to resist them after they are bought.

Opponent Process Theory

Opponent process theory, from the work of Solomon and Corbit (see Solomon, 1980), is a theory of acquired motivation to explain behaviours that are not based on innate needs such as hunger and thirst. This theory centres upon the automatic regulation of emotional states, both pleasant and unpleasant, and, while the theory applies to drinking and drug use, it is not limited to these. It is a theory of emotional or *affective* dynamics which 'assumes that for some reason the brains of all mammals are organized to oppose or suppress many types of emotional arousals or hedonic processes, whether they are pleasurable or aversive, whether they have been generated by positive or negative reinforcers' (p. 698).

There are three basic premises central to opponent process theory. First, that any stimulation is automatically followed by *affective contrast*. Gambling may be used as an example here. In the gambler's early experience, while waiting for the horse to run or the reels on the gaming machine to come to rest, the experience is one of excitement; after the bet is over, there will follow a contrasting feeling of deflation (this may be delayed where the elation is prolonged by winning). The second premise is that of *affective habituation* – with experience, the reaction to a stimulus will lessen. Where the gamblers are concerned, the excitement will lessen as more bets are made. The third premise is that of *affective withdrawal* – that is, the affective after-reaction will grow in intensity and duration and will appear to have the opposite quality to the initial reaction to the stimulus. Our gamblers will not feel the previous levels of excitement when betting, and may even feel depressed. They may attempt to regain the high by raising the stakes, or dispel low moods by spending more time gambling.

Let us look at drug use in terms of opponent process theory. The first use of a drug may be reinforcing through producing a buzz. (The theory allows that if a behaviour is not reinforcing in this primary way, then social pressure may contribute to further use.) Drug use elicits an 'a' process which results in pleasure, called an 'A' state. The theory assumes that the brain is programmed to correct emotional states, both pleasurable and aversive, and so the 'a' process sets off an opponent 'b' process, giving rise to its associated 'B' state, the withdrawal experience.

Over time, the 'b' process becomes stronger; that is, as a person gains experience, the opponent process is set off more quickly and it becomes more powerful. This accounts for the development of tolerance. For example, a regular drug user upon taking the drug will trigger off an opponent process that is quick and strong. This will counteract the effects of the drug, and the experienced user will need to take more of the drug than a novice user to feel the same effects. Of course, as the 'b' process becomes stronger, so does the 'B' state; withdrawal symptoms become more severe. A critical feature in the development of addiction is when the drinker or drug user realizes that he or she can avoid the withdrawal symptoms by drinking or using drugs. The person has acquired a motivation to take drugs based upon the avoidance of unpleasant symptoms; that is, drug use is now negatively reinforced (Shipley, 1987).

It is asserted that the 'a' and 'b' processes can become conditioned to the situation in which they occur. In Chapter 1, Siegel's (1988) experiments with rats were described. Rats who had been given a series of morphine injections showed greater tolerance to the drug, as measured by sensitivity to pain, when they were tested under the same environmental conditions as those in which they had received the drug. That is, tolerance is conditioned to environmental cues. Opponent process theory provides us with a mechanism to explain this phenomenon. Donovan and Chaney (1985) give an example of how conditioned opponent processes would work with a problem drinker. Stimuli associated with the pleasurable 'A' state, for instance a bottle of whisky, would set off the 'a' process which would swiftly be counteracted by the stronger 'b' process resulting in discomfort. This might then lead to relief drinking. Stimuli associated with the unpleasant 'B' state would be aversive in themselves, such as waking up with a hangover, and would lead directly to relief drinking. The non-problem drinker does not have to contend with these strong opponent processes.

The critical issue here in relation to treatment is the 'b' process and the engagement in the addictive behaviour to avoid the unpleasant 'B' state. Since it is the 'a' process that sets off the 'b' process, then it seems that one way to introduce control is through aversion therapy. For drinkers, Donovan and Chaney (1985) suggest that the stimuli surrounding the onset of drinking should be made less pleasant, so that the individual would come to avoid them. As we shall see later, aversion therapy need not mean giving people electric shocks or drugs to make them vomit. These days, less harsh cognitive techniques are more commonly used.

Social Learning Theory

Social learning theory (Bandura, 1977a) may be considered an interactionist theory; that is, the person, the environment and the behaviour all interact with each other to exert influence in all directions. The theory includes concepts derived from classical and operant conditioning, but it moves beyond these to assign importance to 'person factors', particularly cognitions.

A person has the capacity to develop internal cognitive models of experience that serve as guides for decision making and future actions. That is, an individual can *symbolize* experience through thought and language, which allows the capability of *forethought*. A person can think and reason in any situation, weighing up the possible outcomes, and decide what to do for the best. Learning from observation is an important aspect of social learning theory. While we may learn directly from experience, as in classical and operant conditioning, we may also learn from other people's experience. This vicarious capability is called *modelling*, and it is a highly efficient way of learning about complex social behaviour patterns and cultural norms of conduct. Finally, the individual has the capacity for *self-regulation*, whereby information about one's behaviour is compared with an internal standard for that behaviour and any discrepancy between the two is corrected by altering the behaviour, the standard, or both of these.

Central to social learning theory is the notion of *self-efficacy* (Bandura, 1977b). Self-efficacy may be defined as a person's evaluation of his or her competence to perform a task in a specific situation. Efficacy judgments will influence what people choose to do, how much effort they may put into the task, and how long they will persist in the face of obstacles. When self-efficacy is low, that is when a person believes himself or herself to be unable to perform a task successfully, then he or she will feel apprehension and will either avoid the task in question or make little effort to meet the challenge. Conversely, when self-efficacy is high, a person will feel relaxed and will seek out situations in which he or she feels competent; should difficulties arise, he or she will rise to meet the challenge.

Self-efficacy judgments are based on four main sources of information:

1   instruction,
2   observation of others' performance,

3   one's own past performance, and
4   emotional arousal.

That is, to feel competent to perform a task effectively, a person must know what to do, have evidence from others' performance that it can be done, have previous personal experience of success, and feel relaxed enough to do it.

Abrams and Niaura (1987) summarize social learning principles in relation to alcohol use and abuse, which may be applied to substance use in general. Where substance use is concerned, social learning theory suggests that we are instructed in cultural norms, and model the behaviour of parents and peers. Individual differences, such as biological make-up, social skills, and the ability to manage emotions, will interact with socialization influences to determine initial patterns of consumption. Direct experience with substances becomes more important as experimentation continues, for example experiencing positive reinforcement of substance use by facilitation of social interaction, and negative reinforcement by tension reduction. Some people may have deficits in social coping skills or low self-efficacy beliefs, and, for those who have learned that substance use helps them cope in the short term, continued substance use will be likely.

With continued substance use, tolerance to the direct reinforcing effects is acquired, and more of the substance may be needed to achieve the desired effects. Dependence may develop, in which case there is a risk for using the substance to avoid withdrawal effects. The person who is consistently reliant upon substance use to provide short term positive outcomes is likely repeatedly to behave in ways that adversely affect his or her social relationships and environment. For example, repeated unreliability, moodiness or aggression may result in the loss of one's job and the breakdown of one's relationships. It is easy to see how this may be the start of a vicious circle where the heavy drinker or drug user loses his or her social and environmental supports, thus creating stresses which, in turn, lead to further drinking or drug use. This illustrates the interactive element of social learning theory.

Circumstances will, of course, vary from one person to the next. Also, for any one person, as time goes by, biological, psychological and social factors change, and so therefore do the reasons for drinking or drug use. That is, the factors that explain maintenance will differ from the factors that explain initiation. Changes in biological, psychological and social factors can equally account for variations in an individual's substance use at the problematic end of the continuum, such as episodes of heavy use and periods of abstinence or controlled use. Social learning theory is thus able to explain variations in substance use between individuals and within individuals across time and situations.

Approaches to change that derive from this theory relate to teaching the person to recognize the risk factors that precipitate substance use, improving alternative coping skills, and enhancing the person's self-efficacy beliefs so that these alternative skills may be used effectively.

Problem Behaviour Theory

Problem behaviour theory (Jessor and Jessor, 1977) is another interactive, social–psychological framework that has been developed to account for a number of problem behaviours in adolescence. Problem behaviours are defined as those that depart from the social and legal norms of society and include drinking, drug use, smoking, precocious sexual activity and delinquency. Evidently, these behaviours occur in a cluster; that is, involvement in one is associated with involvement in the others. It is interesting to note, by the way, that in the 1970s Jessor included 'activist protest', that is taking part in political marches and demonstrations, within his problem behaviour cluster (Jessor, 1987). This illustrates the point that scientific study is not as unbiased as we would sometimes like to believe; you only find what you look for!

The focus is primarily upon three systems of psychosocial influence: *the personality system, the environment system,* and *the behaviour system.* Within each system there are instigations to problem behaviour and controls against it, and together they produce a state called *proneness* to problem behaviour. Since instigations and controls vary amongst individuals, the degree of proneness to problem behaviour is idiosyncratic. Of fundamental importance is that there are constant changes in each of these systems for any individual, therefore proneness to problem behaviour is not static across time.

Jessor (1987) talks of personality proneness, environmental proneness and behavioural proneness, which combine to generate 'the sovereign explanatory concept in Problem Behavior Theory – *psychosocial proneness*' (p. 332). This psychosocial proneness is synonymous with the concept of *risk*, and we may address ourselves to the study of psychosocial risk factors for problem behaviours.

The degree of proneness to problem behaviours may be seen as lying somewhere on a continuum of *conventionality–unconventionality.*

The conventional profile is that of an adolescent who does not drink, smoke or use drugs; does well at school; goes to church; does not approve of deviance; has controlling but supportive parents; eats his or her greens; gets plenty of fresh air and exercise; and goes to bed early. The unconventional profile is that of an adolescent who drinks, smokes and uses drugs; does not do well at school; does not go to church; hangs around with a bunch of kids that his or her parents do not like; gets into trouble; eats junk food; will not exercise; and comes home late. As Donovan *et al.* (1991) point out, attempts to change any part of that pattern may need to deal with the pattern as a whole. That is, it may be futile to tackle drinking or drug use unless attention is also paid to broader lifestyle issues, such as academic achievement, health and leisure activities.

Expectancy Theory

Expectancy theory, originating from the work of Tolman (1932), is a cognitive theory that is useful in bridging the gap between the individual's past experience and later behaviour (Goldman, 1989). As people grow up, they learn about alcohol and drugs from what they see going on around them and what they are told: they watch what their parents and friends do and listen to what they say; they are given drug education in schools; they see alcohol and drug use on television and in films; they read about alcohol and drug use; they see licit substances advertised; and they are exposed to campaigns against illicit substances. It is hardly surprising, then, that beliefs about alcohol and drugs are held from an early age.

One particular type of belief is known as an *outcome expectancy*. This is the knowledge of the relationship between behaviour and behavioural outcomes; the knowledge that *if* drinking or drug use occurs, *then* a specific outcome will follow. It is this anticipatory 'if–then' relationship between events which is the defining feature of an outcome expectancy. In the case of drug use, outcome expectancies may affect different response systems to create physical, psychological and behavioural changes. Outcome expectancies may link drug use with the physical, psychological or behavioural effects following it in a way that has nothing to do with any pharmacological effect of the drug. For example, being at a party calls for partylike behaviour – chatting, dancing and generally having fun. If the use of a drug, for example alcohol, is also common at parties, then the individual may develop an expectancy that alcohol causes these high spirits. It cannot be assumed that the drug effect is necessary to the behavioural outcome; the outcome expectancy may be the causal factor. Expectancy effects always complicate matters when it comes to looking at the pharmacological effects of drugs (Goldman *et al.* 1987a).

Outcome expectancies relate to specific circumstances. That is, they vary with both the context of drug use and internal cues. For example, as we have seen, a common expectancy is that drinking alcohol at a party leads to high spirits; the same outcome expectancy may not hold for solitary drinking, where it is probably more common to expect alcohol to lead to a maudlin mood. Where internal cues are concerned, expectancies about substance use may relate to tension reduction, mood management and relief of withdrawal symptoms.

Expectancy theory can explain initiation to substance use, since expectancies have been found to exist prior to experience with alcohol and drugs. They may also account for increased substance use, up to addiction levels, through positive outcome expectancies becoming associated with more and more life contexts. This theory is not incompatible with biological theories in that some people may be physiologically unable to tolerate alcohol or drugs and they will not, therefore, develop positive outcome expectancies.

Expectancy theory offers directions for prevention and intervention. Assessment of expectancies may help in the identification of those who are at risk for developing problems later on. In addition, outcome expectancies may be modified in programmes to reduce alcohol and drug use.

Implications of Psychological Approaches to Addiction

There Is No Single Explanation of Addiction

The first major implication of psychological approaches to addiction is that there is no single explanation of addiction. It is clear that a number of factors must be taken into account in explaining addiction. These factors lie within three major domains. *Biological factors* have a part to play through a person being more or less predisposed to develop an addiction by virtue of his or her biological make-up. *Psychological factors* are also important in that any individual will behave in ways which are influenced by his or her personal learning history. Addictive behaviours occur within a *cultural and social context* and issues relating to rules, norms and values are important in explaining addiction.

These systems – biological, psychological and social – *interact* with each other to determine the nature and degree of the addictive behaviour in any person. For example, a person may be biologically prone to excessive alcohol consumption, but live in a society where heavy drinking is frowned upon and is unlikely, therefore, to proceed to problem drinking. Variables from each of the three systems differ from one person to the next, therefore it is important to treat each person as an individual, looking at his or her own unique profile.

Over recent years, an integrative model, called the *biopsychosocial model*, has begun to emerge. This model may serve as a reminder that we have to include information from a number of fields in understanding addiction. In this book, there is acknowledgement throughout that biological factors have a contribution to make. Alcohol and drugs have a physical action upon the body; substances must be metabolized, and metabolism differs from one person to the next; and substances can cause organic damage that affects behaviour. Indeed, it is acknowledged that the psychology of reinforcement and learning has a biological basis in the brain and its neural circuitry. Brain organization differs from one person to the next, and so there is variability in how readily people learn from experience, and in their cognitive abilities such as decision making, problem solving, and forward planning. Similarly, acknowledgement is given to the fact that addictive behaviours are carried out within a broad cultural framework. Politics, economics and the law all play their part in setting the scene for addictive behaviours to occur.

Addicts Are Not Different from the Rest of Us

Psychological theories explain 'normal' as well as 'abnormal' behaviour, and the same principles apply to initiation, maintenance, dependence and change. That is, there is no special subgroup of 'addicts' who are different from the rest of us. In psychological approaches, biological, psychological and social factors are incorporated to explain individual variations in engagement in addictive behaviours. Clearly, one aspect that must be explained is the degree of a person's involvement in the addictive behaviour. That is a person may be an abstainer, a moderate drinker or drug user, or an excessive user. Over a person's life span, there may well be fluctuations in the degree of involvement: from abstinence to moderate use; from moderate use to excessive use; from excessive use to abstinence or moderate use. Psychological theories attempt to explain how these fluctuations occur. The point to note here is that addiction is not necessarily progressive, as the disease model would have us believe. There is a *continuum of levels of involvement* and the individual will slide up and down that continuum depending upon the current situation and his or her skills for coping with that situation. For example, many people will drift in and out of problematic substance use consequent upon finding or losing jobs, being in a stable relationship or breaking up from their partner, and having good living accommodation or finding themselves without a home.

There Is No Cut-off Point for Addiction

The theories presented here do not present us with a cut-off point for addiction. It is acknowledged that people may have problems at any level of consumption, and that these problems may be interpersonal, legal, financial, scholastic, work-related, psychological or physical. There is no absolute cut-off point for addiction at which we may place our level of concern, as the disease model seems to suggest. That is, anyone who is experiencing problems in relation to substance use may be a candidate for help, and we need not label this person an 'alcoholic' or an 'addict' in order to make him or her eligible for our attention.

Addiction Is Not Irreversible

None of the processes suggested by these psychological theories is irreversible. That is, we have moved away from the notion of addiction as a progressive and irreversible disease process. Clearly this has implications for interventions to reduce substance use. Using psychological theories, we can come up with a whole *range of possible goals and interventions*. First of all, we do not have to advocate abstinence in every case; for some people a reduction in substance use will be sufficient, and for others it may be more pressing to teach methods of harm reduction. This latter point is important these days when considering HIV transmission through the sharing of needles by intravenous drug users; it is crucial and urgent to protect against HIV infection and the drug use *per se* takes second place to this.

The theories presented here give indications as to what kinds of intervention may be developed. A few of these have been mentioned, for example cue exposure with response prevention, discrimination training, contingency management, aversion therapy, skills training, lifestyle modification and changing outcome expectancies. Many more interventions based on psychological theories have been developed, and these are currently showing good outcomes. These will be described in Chapter 5 which looks at change in addictive behaviours.

Psychological Theories Are Not Specific to Addictive Behaviours

Finally, psychological theories are not specific to addictive behaviours. The theories presented in this chapter are theories which apply to all kinds of behaviour, not just addictive behaviours. In the study of substance use, the emphasis on biological factors has been reduced; that is, biological factors have been cut down to size, but not completely disregarded. Consequently, mainstream psychological theories have been used to explain drinking and drug use, as they have other behaviours. If all behaviours are explained according to the same principles, then this allows for the inclusion of non-substance-based behaviours as addictions. Gambling and sex have already been mentioned in passing. This actually presents us with a problem in defining what an addiction is, and in deciding to which behaviours the concept can be applied. Can we, as common parlance these days suggests, become addicted to almost anything? Can one become a workaholic, a chocoholic, addicted to love, and so on?

So, What Is Addiction?

Non-substance-based addictions, such as gambling, have often been brought into line with the addiction to substances by reference to the brain's ability to produce its own internal addictive substances (Davies, 1992). Endorphins are opiates produced naturally by the brain in response to high arousal states. J.B. Davies (1992) points out that,

> The idea that people can generate their own internal addictive pharmacology can be applied to all sorts of behaviours other than gambling and drug-taking, including such valued activities as playing the violin, walking to the North Pole, or becoming a Member of Parliament; things which in themselves are not regarded as pathological. Consequently, if we adopt this line of argument, any kind of commitment or dedication stands in danger of becoming an 'addiction', especially if the person feels good as a consequence (p. 73).

If we admit the conclusion that addictive behaviours can be understood by the same principles that apply to any behaviour, 'it is precisely *because* of this understanding that the boundary conditions of addictive behaviours are difficult to establish' (Miller and Brown, 1991, p. 10). Addictive behaviours may be considered as those that meet two criteria. First, they are *motivated by short-term gains*; that is, immediate gratification is more important in determining the behaviour than are the longer term negative consequences. However, this is not sufficient to define addictive behaviours since many behaviours that are motivated by short term gains would not usually be considered addictive, for example sunbathing, stealing or skipping school. These are simply goal-directed behaviours with calculated risks attached (Miller and Brown, 1991). A second definitional criterion of addictive behaviours is that they *involve a degree of diminished control over the behaviour.* Where addictions are concerned, many people express impaired control over their behaviour, and this is clearly a phenomenon that must be explained. Acknowledgement of the phenomenon of diminished control does not imply a return to the disease model of addiction. Psychological explanations of diminished control will be given in Chapter 4.

Of course, to say that a behaviour is addictive is not to say that everyone engaging in that behaviour is addicted to it. As already stated, there are dynamic processes leading to initiation, maintenance, dependence and change. Therefore it makes sense to talk about *addictive behaviours*, those that hold the potential for addiction, and *addiction*, that is a style of involvement in a behaviour characterized by the experience of diminished control.

The actual behaviours that may be included within the addictions field are numerous. In his book *Excessive Appetites*, Orford (1985) includes excessive gambling, overeating and excessive sexuality, in addition to alcohol and drug use. He also mentions a number of other behaviours that he considers relevant, namely kleptomania, fire-setting, overwork, and playing electronic games. It is not, therefore, the behaviour as such that defines an addiction; possibly any behaviour could be addictive under some circumstances. In this book, the focus is primarily upon those behaviours for which there is most consensus regarding their status as addictive – alcohol and drug use. Reference will be made to non-substance-based behaviours to illustrate certain points, but these will be represented less comprehensively in the following chapters, reflecting current biases in the scientific literature.

It has already been stated that for an addiction to develop, one must start in the first place. We must turn now to an investigation of initiation to and maintenance of addictive behaviours.

Chapter 3

Initiation and Maintenance

The origins of drug use surely depended upon the chance discovery that certain plants produced psychoactive effects. This happened so long ago that it remains a matter for the imagination. Ever since those prehistoric days, drug use has acquired a variety of social meanings. Over time, science and social organization interact to change the meaning of drug use in society. Ghodse (1989) illustrates this using coffee as an example. Coffee was known to the Arabs in the sixth century, and used then for its medicinal properties. Coffee-drinking became widespread in the fourteenth century with advent of the technique of roasting and grinding coffee beans. In the Arab world, where alcohol was banned by the Koran, coffee-drinking took on something of the social meaning that alcohol has today in the West; coffee houses were social meeting places. The authorities, however, came to fear that coffee houses were centres of political dissent and social unrest, and moves were made to ban coffee. When prohibition failed, coffee was taxed heavily, providing a source of considerable revenue for the authorities. Coffee drinking spread to Britain in the seventeenth century, to be met with a similar response. Again, coffee houses were seen as centres of political insurrection, and moves were made to close them down. By the end of the eighteenth century, coffee houses began to wane in popularity, and tea became the national drink. Although tea also contains some caffeine, this drink has never acquired the same association with political activism.

This tale of coffee drinking and responses to it highlights some of the major themes relevant to understanding drug use. Many of the illicit drugs we know today were originally used for medicinal purposes, but their use eventually assumed a social meaning. As Ghodse says, drug use can be the whole reason for a group coming together, the drug being the substance of communication and the drug-taking rituals being the group activity. Alcohol use in the West today fulfils a social function in that people meet and relax in pubs and clubs. Illicit drug use fulfils a similar social function in that those who use them meet and share a 'mind-expanding' experience, for example through attendance at all-night 'raves' where taking the drug ecstasy is a central activity.

Drug use and its social meaning is influenced over time by society's responses to it. Legislation to control various substances imposes a certain meaning upon drug use, creating drug-using subcultures with their own special identity. Scientific advances also influence drug use: for example, the manufacture of 'designer drugs', which are new substances to which legislative controls do not apply. Technological advances also have an impact, for example the discovery that cocaine can be converted into 'crack', which may then be heated and the vapour inhaled, giving a more intense 'hit' than snorting cocaine powder (Strang, 1990).

Legislation, science and technology influence fashion where substance use is concerned and the current fashion reflects the social meaning of substance use. Bearing in mind that there is a social meaning to substance use, and remembering that this changes over time, we shall now look at issues relating to taking up substance use.

Obviously, no one can proceed to addiction without beginning somewhere. As we shall see, many young people in western society use alcohol, and quite a number at least try cigarettes, cannabis and other illicit drugs. There is an important purpose in studying initiation to behaviour in the addictions field, since the old adage 'prevention is better than cure' is nowhere more apt than here; if people do not start in the first place, then there is no chance of finding themselves later on in the position of having to seek a 'cure'. Efforts to design effective prevention programmes benefit from the study of the factors involved in initiation to addictive behaviours.

It is perhaps surprising that experimental substance use ever leads on to regular use. We often hear seasoned drinkers say that they had to overcome their initial dislike for the taste of alcohol, and many smokers describe the difficulty they had inhaling the smoke of their first few cigarettes. Cannabis smokers often report feeling very little effect of the drug the first few times they try it, and even heroin users do not always experience a high with their first dose. After initial experimentation, what then motivates people to continue with addictive behaviours?

This chapter is essentially a review of those factors that may be considered to place a person at risk of starting a behaviour that may later develop into an addiction, and the circumstances that contribute to the maintenance of addictive behaviours. Before going on to address these risk factors, it is important to look at prevalence rates of drinking and drug use amongst young people. One issue which requires attention at this point is the main method by which information about drinking and drug use is collected – self-report.

Many researchers who wish to find out about drinking and drug use simply ask people to tell them about their involvement in these behaviours. *Self-report measures,* as they are known, have attracted some criticism in the research field. The validity of self-report has been questioned; that is, how can we be sure that respondents are telling the truth? Some people may wish to conceal the true extent of their drinking and drug use, and others may give inflated estimates to give the impression that they are living in the fast lane. Validity of self-report will be influenced by the conditions under which the information is being collected: who is asking the questions and for what purpose? Researchers can enhance the likelihood of getting valid self-reports by explaining why the information is required, assuring the respondent of confidentiality, and making cross-checks with other sources of information. The importance of these strategies becomes apparent when one understands that information about individual patterns of drinking and drug use are not available from other sources. After all, who knows better about your drinking and drug use than yourself? There is no better source of information, and therefore reliance on self-report is frequently essential.

Prevalence

Swadi (1988) studied substance use in a large sample of London school pupils between 11 and 16 years of age. The information was collected by issuing questionnaires that were completed under examination conditions with assurances of complete confidentiality. The prevalence of substance use for each age group is presented in Table 3.1.

The mean age at which drinkers in this sample reported having their first drink was 11.6 years. Overall, 63 per cent reported having drunk alcohol, with prevalence rates rising from 45 per cent at age 11 years to 80 per cent at age 16 years, and 11 per cent drank once a week or more. Gender differences were very small: 63 per cent of the boys had drunk alcohol at some time or other, and 12 per cent were regular drinkers (i.e. once a week or more); 64 per cent of the girls had drunk alcohol, with 11 per cent being regular drinkers.

Because drinking is not against the law, although there are legal

Table 3.1 *Prevalence of substance use by age (Swadi, 1988)*

	Age in years					
	11 (n = 284)	12 (641)	13 (598)	14 (562)	15 (624)	16 (329)
	Percentage					
Ever used alcohol	45	48	60	69	76	80
Currently smoking cigarettes	5	8	16	26	27	31
Ever used solvents or illegal drugs	13	14	19	24	26	26
Repeated use of solvents or illegal drugs	2	4	5	10	14	16
Ever used hard drugs	2	2	4	8	8	8

Table 3.2 *Prevalence and amounts of drinking from a population census survey (Marsh, et al. 1986)*

		Age in years				
		13	14	15	16	17
		Percentage				
Alcohol users	*Male*	80	88	91	88	91
	Female	74	86	90	85	88
Regular alcohol users	*Male*	29	34	52	46	61
	Female	11	24	37	36	54
*Units**						
Mean weekly alcohol consumption	*Male*	8.3	11.4	15.9	10.6	16.1
	Female	4.7	8.0	9.1	6.2	7.0

*Note: * One unit equals one standard drink equals 8 grammes alcohol*

restrictions, information is relatively easy to collect through population censuses. A national survey by the Office of Population Censuses and Surveys (OPCS) has provided information about the drinking of 4908 adolescents (Marsh *et al.*, 1986). Data are presented in Table 3.2. This survey shows that most adolescents drink at least occasionally. By the age of 17 years, over half drink at least once a week, and while girls are almost as likely to drink as are boys, their alcohol consumption is lower.

Cigarette smoking is far from uncommon. Swadi's study shows that 5 per cent of 11-year-olds smoke, rising to 31 per cent in 16-year-olds. Gender differences are apparent here. Results from Swadi's study, presented in Table 3.3, show that girls are more likely to smoke and smoke daily than are boys.

The mean age at which Swadi's sample reported starting to use any drug was 13 years. Overall, just over 20 per cent of this sample had

Table 3.3   *Cigarette smoking by gender (Swadi, 1988)*

	Boys (n = 1695)	Girls (1378)	Total (3073)
	Percentage		
Occasional smokers	8.1	13.9	10.7
Daily smokers	6.5	9.9	8.0
Total smokers	14.6	23.9	18.7

Table 3.4 *Type of substance, frequency of use, and gender of user (Swadi, 1988)*

		Only once/occasionally	Weekly/daily
Cannabis	Male*	50%	9%
	Female+	48%	7%
Solvents	Male	42%	4%
	Female	53%	12%
Stimulants	Male	14%	2%
	Female	13%	3%
Tranquillizers	Male	11%	0.8%
	Female	14%	0.8%
Cocaine	Male	6%	0.5%
	Female	9%	5%
Hallucinogens	Male	10%	1%
	Female	6%	0.8%
Heroin	Male	4%	3%
	Female	4%	6%

Notes: * n = 377
+ n = 253

used solvents or illicit drugs at least once, with 13 per cent at age 11 years rising to 26 per cent at age 16 years. Information about the type of drug used, the frequency of use, and the gender of the user is presented in Table 3.4. These figures show that cannabis and solvents are by far the most widely used substances, with around half of the sample having at least tried these. Use of other substances is relatively rare. It is interesting to note that girls are significantly more likely to be regular users of solvents and cocaine.

A similar picture emerges from the USA. The National Institute on Drug Abuse conducted a household survey in 1985 and found that, amongst the 12 to 17 year age group, 45 per cent smoked cigarettes, 56 per cent drank alcohol and 30 per cent had tried at least one illicit drug. The most commonly used illicit drug was cannabis, used by 24 per cent, followed by solvents (9 per cent), analgesics (6 per cent), stimulants (6 per cent) and cocaine (5 per cent), with less than 1 per cent ever having used heroin (cited in Newcomb and Bentler, 1989).

Looking at the prevalence figures presented here, we can see that alcohol use is a normal activity amongst young people; experimentation with soft drugs is fairly common; about one-fifth of youngsters smoke cigarettes at least occasionally; but hard drug use is still relatively uncommon. The consequences of hard drug use can be devastating, yet the costs to society in terms of the social and physical consequences of illicit drug use are small when compared to the costs incurred from drinking and smoking. Heavy drinking is strongly associated with a range of serious social problems, including crime, relationship problems and absenteeism from work, as well as injury from accidents and health problems. Few people these days would deny the physical damage caused by cigarette smoking – lung cancer, heart disease and respiratory ailments. Given the prevalence rates of drinking and smoking, it is proper that concern should surround these activities.

This serves to highlight the importance of studying the factors involved in the use of substances of all kinds, licit and illicit. Although it may seem obvious, where all of these behaviours are concerned 'use is a necessary antecedent to abuse' (Newcomb and Bentler, 1989, p. 244) and it is, therefore, important to understand the factors that influence initiation to substance use.

Risk Factors

A list of factors which determine behaviour was presented in Table 2.1. These were the cultural context, family factors, peer influences, factors relating to the person's lifestyle and environmental circumstances, behavioural skills, thoughts, feelings and physical factors. Those factors that are of particular relevance to taking up addictive behaviours will be addressed under five headings:

1 *Legal issues*, since, where substance use is concerned, this is one aspect of the cultural context with significant influence.
2 *Family influences* are important particularly in terms of modelling, attitudes and management practices.
3 *Peer influences* are commonly credited with considerable power to influence a young person's behaviour.
4 *Behavioural factors* are also important, given the observation that drinking and drug use occur in a cluster with other problem behaviours as part of a deviant or unconventional lifestyle.

5   Finally, *psychological factors* play their part in initiation to and maintenance of addictive behaviours, and attention will be paid to issues relating to thoughts and feelings.

Each of the five areas listed above will be considered in turn in this chapter. Before going on to describe risk factors within the framework of these broad areas, it is important to note that there is an interaction between the individual and his or her structural and social environment that determines whether or not a substance is used, the type of substance used, and the extent of use of any substance (Davis and Tunks, 1991). That is, although risk factors are neatly separated out for the purposes of this chapter, there is in reality a complex interrelationship amongst factors, and it is important to look at the whole picture in explaining why any particular person begins to use any substance and why some people go on to problematic substance use.

Legal Issues

Many behaviours are to some degree controlled by the rules of the culture in which we live. All of the substances mentioned above are subject to control by the law, including restrictions on possession, sale and supply.

In Britain, where alcohol is concerned, it is against the law to give intoxicating liquor to a child under 5 years old, except on medical orders. Apart from this, young people under 18 years of age may consume alcohol quite lawfully, except in licensed premises and in certain areas of the country where there are by-laws prohibiting drinking in public places. A person of age 14 years may enter licensed premises, but may not consume or purchase alcohol; at age 16 years, drinking beer or cider is permitted in dining areas of licensed premises. Only at age 18 years is the purchase and consumption of alcohol on licensed premises unrestricted. It is an offence for a licensee or staff of licensed premises knowingly to sell alcohol to a person under the age of 18 years (and, incidentally, to any person who is drunk).

Smoking is not against the law at any age, but the Children and Young Persons (Protection from Tobacco) Act (1991) forbids retailers from selling tobacco products to anyone under the age of 16 years. While the use of solvents is a cause of considerable concern, it again is not in itself an offence against the law. It is, however, an offence to supply any volatile substance to a person under the age of 18 years where the supplier believes that it will be used for the purpose of causing intoxication (Gossop, 1993).

In the UK, drugs are controlled principally by the Misuse of Drugs Act (1971). This states the requirements for prescription, safe custody and record keeping, as well as defining offences relating to production, cultivation, supply and possession of drugs (Ghodse, 1989). The act classifies drugs into three categories: *Class A* includes cocaine, heroin, LSD, methadone, morphine and opium; *Class B* includes amphetamines, barbiturates and cannabis; *Class C* includes appetite suppressants and sedatives. The penalties for offences involving controlled drugs are most severe for Class A drugs and trafficking is more severely punished than is possession.

Medical professionals must abide by the Misuse of Drugs Regulations (1985), which state who is authorized to possess and supply controlled drugs, and rules governing prescription (Ghodse, 1989). These regulations also oblige a doctor to notify the Chief Medical Officer at the Home Office of a patient suspected to be addicted to certain controlled drugs, including cocaine, heroin, methadone, morphine and opium.

Looking back at the prevalence rates of substance use amongst young people, it is clear to see that permitted substances, that is alcohol, cigarettes and solvents, are those most commonly used. Obviously, the legal situation affects the availability of any substance. Alcohol, for example, is readily available to most young people in the home, pubs and shops. By contrast, illicit drugs are harder to obtain. Nonetheless, young people do manage to get hold of illicit drugs, but only some go out of their way to do so. Factors relating to availability are only part of the story.

Family Influences

Families influence initiation to substance use in a number of ways. Leaving aside for the moment issues relating to genetic transmission which will be covered in the next chapter, factors to do with modelling, parenting practices, and family cohesion deserve attention.

Brook *et al.* (1986) conducted a longitudinal study of junior high school students over two years. At the start of the study, their sample contained 318 non-drinkers; after two years 155 had tried alcohol and

22 were regular drinkers. Family factors were studied, amongst others, to identify correlates of initiation to alcohol use. First, initiates in comparison to non-initiates reported *greater use of drugs by family members*, both parents and siblings. Drug use here includes legal substances such as alcohol and prescribed drugs, as well as illicit drugs. This indicates that direct imitation of family members, or modelling, is an important determinant of the adolescent's drinking. Second, permissiveness on the part of the parents was associated with increased initiation to drinking. This shows that *parental tolerance or approval* of drinking is a significant predictor of the amount of alcohol consumed by adolescents.

A similar situation pertains to the onset of illicit drug use, in that parental use is associated with initiation to use in adolescents (Kandel *et al.*, 1978). Conrad *et al.* (1992), in their review of studies related to the onset of smoking, noted that parental behaviour and approval for smoking played a less significant role here than expected.

Another important issue is that of *family management*. McKay *et al.* (1991) examined family functioning and substance use in 45 adolescents in psychiatric treatment. Adolescents who drank heavily were more likely to come from unemotional families where members' roles were not clear. Marijuana use, on the other hand, was associated only with lack of role clarity, that is where there is confusion about who is supposed to be doing what. Hawkins *et al.* (1992), in their excellent review of risk factors for adolescent substance use, conclude that

> the risk of drug abuse appears to be increased by family management practices characterized by unclear expectations for behavior, poor monitoring of behavior, few and inconsistent rewards for positive behavior, and excessively severe and inconsistent punishment for unwanted behavior. (p. 83)

Hawkins *et al.* (1992) also mention *low bonding to the family* as a risk factor. Bonding to the family may protect against initiation to substance use because engagement in family activities will leave less time for association with peers and will encourage the internalization of conventional norms and behaviours. *Family conflict* may also play a part in initiation to substance use. Baer *et al.* (1987) studied 425 junior high school students and found that the more family conflict they identified, the greater was the level of alcohol use. They do, however, point out that family conflict is much less powerful than parental modelling and peer influences in predicting adolescent alcohol use.

To summarize, family factors that place an adolescent at risk for drinking and drug use include parental modelling of substance use, tolerance or approval of substance use, unclear rules for behaviour, inconsistent rewards and punishments, low family bonding and high levels of family conflict. There are, however, factors outside the family environment that impact upon drinking and drug use, most notably the influence of peers.

Peer Influences

Peer influence is widely assumed to affect drinking and drug use amongst adolescents. While it has been noted that drinkers and drug users associate more with other drinkers and drug users, the similarities could be due to one of two processes: socialization or selection. Under *socialization*, similarity develops as a result of interpersonal influence or 'peer pressure'. *Selection*, on the other hand, is where the behaviour in question, in this case substance use, exists prior to the friendship and adolescents choose to mix with others who are similar to themselves, who are also substance users.

A longitudinal study by Downs (1987), where drinking by subjects and their peers was measured, indicates that there is a reciprocal relationship; that is the subjects under study influenced their friends to drink as much as their friends influenced them. This reciprocal relationship held true only for close friends and not the wider circle, which goes some way to dispelling the view of the passive adolescent reacting to the pressures exerted by an amorphous peer group.

Kandel (1985) reports similarities in illicit drug use between adolescent best friends; where marijuana is concerned, a non-user is most likely to have a best friend who is also a non-user, and a user is most likely to have a best friend who is a user. Further studies of the making and breaking of friendships across time showed that, where marijuana use was concerned, similarity predicted not only the choice of friend, but also the continuation of the friendship. Where dissimilarity arose, the adolescent would either break off the friendship or modify his or her behaviour to re-establish congruity. That is, selection and socialization both play their part in friendship. As a reminder of the importance of selection, Kandel points out that her results suggest that 'estimates of peer influence are inflated, since they fail to take into account the role of prior similarity in friendship formation' (p. 157).

Of course, not all peer groups promote drug use. Kandel (1985) notes that gregarious adolescents can belong to a drug using group or a non-drug using group, and drug use depends upon membership of a group whose members use drugs. Kandel's comment is that belonging to a peer group does not in itself mean that an adolescent is necessarily going to be antagonistic to adults and their conventions; there can be continuity of values across the generations.

The Relative Influence of Parents and Peers

A considerable amount of research has been conducted on the relative influence upon adolescents' drinking and drug use of parents and peers. Parents and peers seem to exert differential influence for different types of drug and at different phases of drug use. Parents play a stronger role in the initiation to alcohol use, while peers play the more important role in the maintenance phase. Peers have the greater influence over both initiation to and maintenance of illicit drug use (Kandel, 1985). Overall, parents have an early influence in modelling substance use behaviour and teaching values relating to alcohol and drugs. Once substance use begins, peers become the dominant social influence and parents exert an influence only indirectly, for example by controlling an adolescent's social activities and timekeeping. Of course, one can choose one's friends and an adolescent may select friends who will reinforce those behaviours in which he or she has decided to engage.

Familial and peer risk factors are also seen to exacerbate each other, such that where familial risks exist then an adolescent is more susceptible to peer risk factors (Brook *et al.*, 1986). However, parental influence appears to have a longer lasting impact than peer influence. Friendships often change rapidly over the course of adolescence, and their effects are relatively transitory compared to parental influences (Kandel, 1985).

Behavioural Factors

Problem behaviour theory (Jessor and Jessor, 1977), described in Chapter 2, showed us that a number of so-called *deviant behaviours*

Table 3.5 *Deviant behaviours that occur in a cluster*

Drinking
Smoking
Illicit drug use
Rebelliousness
Delinquency
Dangerous driving
Aggression
Poor academic achievement
Less church attendance
Less orientation to work
Early sexual intercourse
Unprotected sex

are likely to co-occur in an individual. Many researchers have identified this cluster, elements of which are presented in Table 3.5.

Longitudinal research indicates a developmental sequence starting with delinquency, progressing to drinking alcohol and smoking cigarettes, then on to smoking marijuana, moving onto problem drinking, and finally using hard drugs. Before investigating this further, an important point must be made about this developmental sequence; where substance use is concerned, while there is a progression, it is not an inevitable progression. Newcomb and Bentler (1989) describe the situation succinctly when they say 'involvement at one stage does not necessarily lead to involvement at the next stage; rather, involvement at the next stage is unlikely without prior involvement in the previous stage' (p. 244). A heroin user, for example, probably started out his or her illicit drug career by using marijuana, but by no means is every marijuana user going to become a heroin user.

Webb *et al.* (1991) studied 114 junior high school students over a period of one year. At the start of the study, none of these youngsters had drunk alcohol, but after the year had passed 48 per cent were drinkers. A number of factors were measured to determine which were associated with the onset of drinking. Involvement in deviant behaviour proved strongly associated, that is those who became drinkers were more likely to be engaged in the cluster of problem behaviours noticed by Jessor and Jessor (1977). Because the young people in this study were abstainers at the start, we may conclude that these risk factors were present before the onset of drinking and not caused by drinking. Brook *et al.* (1986), in their longitudinal study, also found that initiation to drinking is associated with unconventionality or nonconformity, that is less orientation to work, tolerance of deviance, and involvement in delinquent behaviours.

In their longitudinal study of 1725 adolescents, Elliott *et al.* (1985) found that delinquency and involvement in delinquent peer groups predicted both later delinquency and illicit drug use. This means that delinquency tends to persist from early to late adolescence, and that delinquency is evident prior to drug use. Brook *et al.* (1989), also in a longitudinal study, found that unconventionality predicted drug use better in younger adolescence compared with later adolescence. This means that unconventionality plays a more important role in early use, and that once drug use has started unconventionality becomes less important and drug use takes on its own influence.

Substance use forms part of an overall unconventional behaviour pattern. It is easy to understand that non-conforming or rebellious children select each other as friends and thereafter a reciprocal inter-personal influence occurs. The use of alcohol and cigarettes prior to illicit substances may be explained in terms of their availability. Once the rewards of drinking and smoking are experienced, the adolescent may feel an attraction toward other substances. For those already in-volved with delinquent peers, the barriers are relatively easy to surmount. Conversely, non-delinquent adolescents are protected against initiation to drug use by being involved in conventional activities, such as studying, playing sport and going to church.

The observation that a number of problem behaviours consistently occur together gives rise to the possibility that there may be a common factor underpinning the entire cluster. One proposal is that there is an underlying disturbance in the regulation of arousal (Miller and Brown, 1991). Zuckerman (1979) suggests that there may be an underlying disposition for *sensation seeking.* This is defined as 'the need for varied, novel, and complex sensations and experiences and the willingness to take physical and social risks for the sake of such experiences' (Zuckerman, 1979, p. 10). People who enjoy arousing experiences will be more likely to use alcohol and drugs, as well as involve themselves in a range of other so-called reckless behaviours. Arnett (1992) mentions drunk driving, dangerous driving, having unprotected sex and antiso-cial behaviour as all related to sensation seeking. Much effort has been directed towards identifying the biological basis of sensation seeking, and relationships have been found with brain wave activity, biochemi-cal activity and sex hormone levels (Arnett, 1992).

Windle (1991) studied the relationship between *difficult tem-perament* and substance use in high school students. The characteris-tics of a difficult temperament are irregular sleeping and eating habits, inflexibility to changes in the environment, high levels of distractibility and low levels of persistence in tasks or activities. Windle found that the greater the number of difficult temperament factors shown by an adolescent, the more likely was that adolescent to use cigarettes, alcohol, marijuana and hard drugs. A difficult temperament in adolescence was associated with hyperactivity and conduct disorder in childhood. In addition to the use of drugs, this difficult temperament in adolescence was associated with depressive symptoms, delinquency and low perceived levels of family support. It is possible, of course, that the manifestation of a difficult temperament may contribute to negative social interactions with parents, teachers and peers. Poor relationships with others may, in turn, lead to poor psychosocial adjustment, and to substance use as a means of coping with problems.

In summary, alcohol and drug use often occur as part of a cluster of problem behaviours. In terms of risk, engagement in one problem behaviour presents a risk for engagement in other kinds of problem behaviour. In particular, delinquency and belonging to delinquent peer groups are significant risk factors for substance use. A connection amongst these problem behaviours may be based in an underlying disposition, such as sensation seeking or difficult temperament, with a biological basis. While the individual may be prone to drinking or drug use as a consequence of a particular disposition, this does not negate the fact that behaviour is instrumental. That is, internal dispositions may play a part in alcohol and drug use, but these must be balanced against the social and psychological consequences of these behaviours in terms of establishing independence from parents, gaining peer acceptance and approval and coping with emotions.

Psychological Factors

We saw in Chapter 2 that *outcome expectancies* have a role to play in substance use. That is, the effects a person expects from drinking or drug use will go some way to determining whether or not the behaviour occurs. Expectancies may be understood as the cognitive channels through which social influences exert their effects.

One important question is how expectancies lead young people to drink or use drugs in the first place. To study this in relation to drinking, Goldman *et al.* (1987c) developed their Alcohol Expectancy Questionnaire – Adolescent Form (AEQ-A). Items contained in this questionnaire require a response of either true or false. Example items are: Drinking alcohol makes the future seem brighter; People feel sexier after a few drinks; Drinking alcohol loosens people up; People do stupid, strange, or silly things when they drink alcohol. Analysis of data collected using this questionnaire shows that it contains seven factors. Alcohol is expected to produce:

1 global positive changes;
2 changes in social behaviour;
3 improved cognitive and motor abilities;
4 sexual enhancement;
5 cognitive and motor impairment;
6 increased arousal; and
7 relaxation and tension reduction.

These seven expectancy factors have been called 'the seven dwarves' by Leigh (1989); after drinking, people expect to become happy, sleepy, dopey, and so on!

Using this questionnaire, Christiansen *et al.* (1982) studied 12 to 19-year-olds and found that alcohol-related expectancies were present prior to drinking experience. As already mentioned in Chapter 2, children receive messages about drinking from parents, peers and the media. They know about alcohol and its effects long before they are of an age to start drinking. Christiansen *et al.* (1989) studied alcohol-related expectancies and the development of drinking in young people in a longitudinal study over the course of one year, beginning when subjects were between the ages of 11 and 14 years. Alcohol-related expectancies measured at the start predicted drinking one year later; the more positive expectancies a young person holds, the more likely is he or she to become a drinker. The best predictors were Factor 2, that alcohol changes social behaviour, and Factor 3, that alcohol improves cognitive and motor abilities. Obviously, these tap two major areas of insecurity common in adolescence – concerns about fitting in, and concerns about being able to do things as well as everyone else. As an aside, it is interesting to note that advertisements for alcohol commonly capitalize on these two insecurities. One advertisement for a brand of white rum shows a group of extraordinarily attractive young people having what is clearly a great time together in the Caribbean. Drink rum and you will be part of the in-crowd seems to be the message. Another advertisement portrays a drinker with superhuman skills, and we can bet he drinks the particular brand of beer that is being promoted.

In summary, research suggests that expectancies that develop during childhood will set the scene for later drinking. Children who expect positive effects from alcohol are more likely to drink, and drink more

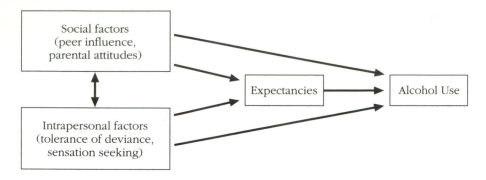

Figure 3.1   *The relationship among social factors, intrapersonal factors, expectancies and alcohol use (after Webb et al. 1993)*

heavily, than those who expect less in the way of positive effects. Expectancies are, therefore, useful in understanding how social influences come to have their effect upon behaviour. However, as for internal dispositions mentioned in the previous section, one cannot ignore the direct social and psychological consequences of drinking and drug use. Webb *et al.* (1993) studied the relationship amongst social factors (peer influence and parental attitudes), intrapersonal factors (tolerance of deviance and sensation seeking), alcohol expectancies and alcohol use. While expectancies played an important mediating role between both social factors and drinking, and intrapersonal factors and drinking, both social factors and intrapersonal factors also exerted a direct influence on drinking. This relationship is represented diagrammatically in Figure 3.1. This means that drinking is determined directly by its consequences (as in operant conditioning theory) and also through mediating cognitive variables (as in expectancy theory).

Another set of risk factors for substance abuse may be given the broad label of *psychological distress*. For example, Baer *et al.* (1987), in their study of junior high school students mentioned above, found that alcohol use was greater in adolescents who reported more stressful life events. The type of life events measured in the study are shown in Table 3.6. These stressors have a greater impact upon adolescents than upon adults, possibly because adolescents have less personal control over them.

Jessor (1987) reports low self-esteem as predictive of involvement in problem behaviours, although findings here are equivocal. Van Hasselt *et al.* (1993) found no differences between adolescent substance abusers and a normative sample on self-esteem, but they did find substance abusers to be more depressed.

Table 3.6   *Stressful life events (after Baer et al., 1987)*

Breaking up with a boyfriend or girlfriend
Change in number of arguments with parents
Beginning to date
Change in number of arguments between parents
Death of someone close
Change in parents' financial status
Move to a new school
Hospitalization of self or family member
Failing a grade in school
Pregnancy in the immediate family
Parents' separation or divorce
New adult included in the family

Table 3.7   *Risk factors for substance use in decreasing order of importance (after Newcomb et al., 1986)*

1 Peer drug use
2 Deviance
3 Perceived drug use by adults
4 Early alcohol use
5 Sensation seeking
6 Poor relationship with parents
7 Low religiosity
8 Poor academic achievement
9 Psychological distress
10 Poor self-esteem

Relative Importance of Risk Factors

Newcomb *et al.* (1986) conducted a longitudinal study of risk factors and substance abuse in high school students. They examined the relative impact of 10 risk factors on the use of a whole range of substances. These factors are presented in Table 3.7 in decreasing order of importance as predictors of drug use.

A number of studies, including the one cited above by Newcomb *et al.*, have shown, however, that it is not *what* the risk factors are, but *how many* there are for an individual to contend with that is most important in predicting substance use. Bry *et al.* (1982) studied six risk factors in relation to drug and alcohol use. These risk factors are shown in Table 3.8. They found a highly significant relationship between the number of risk factors and the extent of substance use; the more risk factors present, the greater the involvement in drug and alcohol use.

Table 3.8   *Risk factors for substance use (Bry et al., 1982)*

Poor school grades
No affiliation with a religion
Under 13 years of age at first independent (i.e. outside family) use of alcohol
High level of psychological distress
Low level of self-esteem
Perception of lack of parental love

These views are endorsed by Farrell *et al.* (1992); in a large scale study of the association between risk factors and substance use in adolescents, they too found a relationship between the total number of risk factors and current use of cigarettes, alcohol, marijuana and other drugs. This suggests that adolescents become involved in substance use for a number of reasons, and that everyone has a unique risk profile.

Implications of Risk

Jessor (1992) poses the question 'What does "at risk" really mean?' and points out that 'at risk' can have two different meanings. First, for those adolescents not yet involved in problem behaviours, there is the risk of becoming involved. Second, for adolescents already involved in problem behaviours, the risks are those of health and life-compromising outcomes.

For the first group, prevention programmes are all-important so that the likelihood of initiation to problem behaviours, including substance use, is minimized. Jessor (1992) notes that 'many adolescents who seem to be at high risk nevertheless do not succumb to risk behavior, or get less involved in it than their peers, or, if involved, seem to abandon it more rapidly than others do' (p. 385). He suggests that it is useful to think not only in terms of risk factors, but also in terms of *protective factors*, which are characteristics or conditions which operate to mitigate risk.

Protective factors include a cohesive family, social controls, peer models for conventional behaviour, a high value on academic achievement, intolerance of deviance and a positive temperament. It seems unclear at present whether protective factors are simply the opposite or the low end of risk factors, or whether these are two separate constructs. However, we do know that the existence of protective factors can offset risk factors. For example, Brook *et al.* (1989) found that academic achievement in adolescence offset the risk for substance use in young people with an angry temperament. That is, youngsters with this angry disposition were highly likely to engage in substance use *except* where they became involved in their school work. Prevention programmes may operate to minimize risk, but they may also address enhancement of protective factors. Approaches to prevention will be described in Chapter 6.

For those adolescents already involved in problem behaviours, the risks are those of getting into trouble with the law, having accidents, getting pregnant, dropping out of school, damaging their health, and so on. For this group, intervention to reduce substance use and associated problems is appropriate. Interventions are covered in Chapter 5.

However, as we have already seen, a fair number of adolescents are involved in substance use to some degree, yet relatively few of them are destined to become dependent on alcohol or drugs. Why do some users become addicted while other do not? For further information on this point, we must look to longitudinal studies which trace *careers* with substance use.

Careers with Substance Use

Addiction is not an inevitable consequence of substance use. The typical pattern is for substance use to peak in late teens or early twenties, and decline thereafter. This pattern is also apparent for delinquent behaviours. The study of the different routes people take over time helps us to understand the different personal, social and environmental factors that play a part in increasing or decreasing use over time.

We know that most adolescents drink, and studies show that drinking can cause problems for young people. Werch *et al.* (1987) studied 410 college students and found that, as alcohol consumption increased, so did the number of problems experienced. Specific problems were noticed at different levels of consumption: light drinkers experienced more illness, such as hangovers, nausea and vomiting; moderate drinkers showed more problems with school and friendships; and heavy drinkers were more likely to get into trouble with the police.

Despite these problems, longitudinal studies show that those who start drinking are unlikely to stop. In fact Johnson (1988) observed that negative consequences were *positively* related to continued use in adolescence. It seems that those consequences labelled 'negative' by researchers may, in fact, be reinforcers for young people's drinking. Becoming noisy and aggressive may be desirable outcomes for the young drinker, particularly in terms of the social kudos some groups attach to these excesses. Apocryphal tales of large quantities of lager consumed, followed by throwing up on the police officer's shoes, can contain an element of bragging.

Nonetheless, we also know that heavy drinking in adolescence is *not* predictive of later problems. Population surveys show that alcohol consumption is highest in the 18 to 24 year age group (Goddard and Ikin, 1989); this indicates that consumption reduces as people get older. Grant *et al.* (1988) have followed a large number of subjects since 1979, finding that drinking typically increases between the ages of 17 and 22 years, but declines thereafter. Andersson and Magnusson (1988) conducted a longitudinal study of boys from school age into adulthood. They found that the frequency of drunkenness in early adolescence was not a good predictor of who may or may not be registered for alcohol abuse in early adulthood. That is, even the most drunkenness-prone teenage boys were unlikely to have serious problems in later life. In conclusion, although few adolescents will stop drinking, most adolescents grow out of problem drinking.

Kandel and Raveis (1989) studied cessation of marijuana and cocaine use in a longitudinal study of men and women identified as users. Over the course of four years, starting when the subjects were aged around 24 years, 34 per cent of men and 45 per cent of women gave up marijuana, and 49 per cent of men and 56 per cent of women gave up cocaine.

It seems, then, that many people moderate their drinking and drug use in their twenties. Why do some people cut down or give up, and why do others not do so? Midanik *et al.* (1990) studied drinkers over a five-year period. Those who changed from being lighter to heavier drinkers, compared with those who remained light drinkers, were reported to be younger, male, less likely to be married, smokers, and experienced more nervousness, depression and emotional trouble. Drinking to cope with personal problems appears to be particularly important in explaining continuation of heavy drinking. Thompson (1989), in a longitudinal study of adolescents, noticed that heavy drinking created disharmony with peer groups, particularly amongst those who drank for non-social purposes. This suggests that those who have personal problems may drink to alleviate them, but that drinking may serve to exacerbate these problems by alienating friends.

In relation to illicit drug use, Kandel and Raveis (1989), again in a longitudinal study, found that those who gave up illicit drug use were more likely to have married and become parents, to have ceased delinquent activities and disengaged from drug-using friends, and to have become religious. These quitters were also more likely to have used drugs socially in the past, whereas non-quitters reported more personal reasons for drug use. Similarly, Brook *et al.* (1989) found, in their longitudinal study of adolescents, that management of psychological distress increased in importance as a factor predicting drug involvement as adolescents grew older. That is, experimental drug use begins as part of the cluster of deviant behaviours, but comes to take on a different purpose as experience with drug use grows – drugs may come to be used to cope with personal problems.

In summary, young adulthood is the time of life when people begin to assume the responsibilities of adulthood – work, marriage and parenthood. These responsibilities contribute to the withdrawal of many young people from their drug-using social groups, abandonment of delinquent activities, and increased involvement in conventional social activities. Lifestyle changes alter the balance of rewards and punishments available in a person's life. Consequently, alcohol consumption is likely to fall from previous levels and illicit drug use is likely to cease.

However, for some people, notably those who use alcohol and drugs to manage psychological distress, there is a likelihood that drinking and drug use will continue. It is amongst this group that we will probably find those who go on to become dependent upon alcohol and drugs. The next chapter addresses issues relating to dependence.

Chapter 4

Dependence

In a psychological analysis of addictive behaviours, it remains important to explain the phenomena underpinning the concept of dependence. In general terms, dependence is often seen as the condition where there is heavy involvement in the addictive behaviour, whether this be drinking, drug-taking, gambling or some other activity. In most cases, this heavy involvement has developed gradually, beginning with occasional indulgence and, with the development of tolerance, rising to the point of excessive indulgence. With excessive indulgence, many problems may arise, yet satisfying the addiction remains a major goal in life despite the costs. These costs are often enormous in terms of loss of home, jobs, relationships, health and even life itself. Control over the addictive behaviour is very difficult, and attempts to stop or cut down are thwarted by unpleasant physical withdrawal symptoms and preoccupation with thoughts about the addictive behaviour. Relapse to the addictive behaviour is common. The person is said to be 'addicted' to or 'dependent' upon the substance or activity of his or her addiction.

This description identifies the key features of dependence: heavy involvement in an addictive behaviour, with persistence in spite of consequent problems; the development of tolerance; engagement in the behaviour to relieve withdrawal symptoms; a sense of compulsion to engage in the behaviour; and diminished control over the behaviour. Before going on to examine these phenomena in greater detail, it must be pointed out that dependence is not a state that may be judged without prejudice.

Orford (1985) puts forward the view that dependence has meaning only where there is pressure to cut down or give up the addictive behaviour. These pressures may be social in origin, for example the pressure to conform to group norms, or they may be self-generated, for example beliefs about how one should behave. The fact of such pressure to give up, and not give in to, addictive behaviours, implies a value attached to moderation. As Saunders and Allsop (1991) point out:

> The Protestant ethic of delayed gratification, the demand for industrial efficiency, disapproval of non-conformity, and condemnation of drug use are all bound up in ideas of self-control and the addiction behaviours . . . Setting standards against which other people's behaviour is to be assessed is a task fraught with risk. There is a potential in such action for a mean-streaked morality, a narrow conservatism of moderation in all things to creep into the frame. Emphasis on self-control can become a demand that we all act in the manner that some self-appointed arbiter believes is desirable. (pp. 283–4)

Who is to say how much is too much? In relation to 'alcoholism', Dylan Thomas shrewdly observed that 'an alcoholic is someone you don't like who drinks more than you do'. It could be argued that everyone has the right to drink freely as long as no harm is caused to others, although since there are medical guidelines about the limits of alcohol consumption above which physical harm becomes increasingly likely (14 units per week for women; 21 units per week for men), one could hold the position that the burden of health costs 'harm' the health service and the tax payer. A similar argument may be applied to other addictive behaviours.

Pressure to cut down or give up can be applied even where indulgence in an addictive behaviour is moderate. A person who has one drink at exactly the same time each evening and has difficulty forgoing the pleasure may be labelled 'addicted'. Assuming that this drinker is experiencing no alcohol-related problems, it is hard to see what might motivate him or her to give up. The pressure to do so arises from others' beliefs that behaviour ought to be flexible and that it does not do to acquire bad habits. Good habits, for example brushing one's teeth every night, do not attract the addiction label. Similarly, solitary drinking is viewed by some as a 'bad sign'. Why is it that a single person should be expected to refrain from pleasures permitted to others who are more gregarious? Such a view may stem from the observation that 'alcoholics' drink all the time, whether they are alone or in company. The reasoning that, since 'alcoholics' drink alone, therefore solitary drinkers are 'alcoholics' is not logical. It is akin to saying that, since people with brain tumours have headaches, anyone with a headache has a brain tumour.

Judgments about costs and benefits are also value-laden. Who is to say that, for example, jobs, homes and relationships are worth guarding, and that placing them in jeopardy by drinking, taking drugs, gambling and the like is foolhardy? Saunders and Allsop (1991) comment that

> When beset . . . by a history of familial discord, poor housing, disrupted relationships, low grade employment or joblessness, plus a poor quality of everyday existence, perhaps the surprise is not that some people fail to regulate themselves well, but that most people do exercise some control, most of the time. (p. 285)

Work, domestic comfort and close personal relationships may not be available to some people, and may not be important to others.

Issues relating to control must, however, be addressed. Heather (1991) notes that a feeling of being 'out of control' is one of the most prominent complaints made by many clients in treatment for addiction, and that an expressed desire to moderate substance use, along with great difficulty in being able to do so, is an experience which cannot simply be dismissed. That is, while issues relating to control are undoubtedly affected by moral judgments, the phenomenon remains. As Heather (1991) puts it:

> it seems highly unlikely that the experience of loss of control was somehow invented as a by-product of the Industrial Revolution . . . Before the 'discovery' of addiction at the end of the eighteenth century, the experience of not being in complete control may not have been expressed in the same language but it is surely difficult to accept that no one ever drank much more than they had originally intended or started to drink when they had promised themselves not to. (p. 154)

He says that 'a satisfactory account of the phenomena denoted by loss of control remains central to a proper understanding of problem drinking and other addictive behaviours' (p. 154).

Heavy involvement in an addictive behaviour, tolerance, withdrawal, compulsion and diminished control are all clinically observed phenomena. That is, certain people can be seen to experience them, or can tell you that they have these experiences. How then, may they be explained? In disease model terms, they are the defining features of dependence, which leads to a tautology. For example, an 'addict' may say he or she craves the object of his or her addiction, and may be observed to indulge that craving by engaging in the addictive behaviour. Craving and loss of control are, thus, terms used to *describe* the person's behaviour. However, in order to *explain* these observations of craving and loss of control, the person is 'diagnosed' as *dependent* upon the

Table 4.1   *Pay-off matrix (after Heather, 1991)*

	Continue	Stop
Benefits	A	B
Costs	C	D

Behaviour will continue if (A + D) > (B + C)

object of the addiction. Since the observations of craving and loss of control have been used to define dependence in the first place, the label 'dependent' does nothing more than summarize these observations – there is no explanation of the observed behaviours attached to the 'diagnosis'.

The task in this chapter is to look more closely at the central features of dependence and provide a psychological explanation for them. In order to organize the material in this chapter, it is necessary to establish a working definition of dependence. Bearing in mind what has been said in the introduction, it seems uncontroversial to define two key issues. First, dependence implies *excessive indulgence* in a behaviour, along with pressure to cease or moderate that behaviour. Second, when the immoderate person attempts to change, it becomes evident that there is *diminished control* over the behaviour. That is, restraint leads to unpleasant feelings, and thoughts about the behaviour begin to dominate one's consciousness, which make change difficult. This chapter will, therefore, be organized in two sections: excessive indulgence and diminished control.

Excessive Indulgence

Some investigators hold that the degree of dependence simply corresponds to the level of involvement in the addictive behaviour. One way to explain engagement in any behaviour is quite simply to look at the positive outcomes balanced against the negative outcomes. Orford (1985) suggests that there is a balance between inclination and restraint dependent upon the ensuing costs and benefits. The situation is summarized in terms of a pay-off matrix by Heather (1991). As we can see from Table 4.1, this is a four-way matrix, balancing the benefits from continuing the behaviour and the costs of stopping, against the benefits of stopping and the costs of continuing. From this matrix, it can be supposed that the behaviour will continue if the total value of cells A plus D exceeds the value of cells B plus C.

Orford (1985) makes two points about costs and benefits. The first is that the balance differs from one person to the next, and varies for any one individual across time. This has already been stated in Chapter 2, where the varying influences of culture, family, social groups and personal factors were acknowledged. The second point made by Orford is that while increased costs may make for increased restraint, the balance is not quite that simple. The complexity may be illustrated using the example of a drinker. The basic problem may be a feeling of sexual inadequacy, and drinking may help alleviate that anxiety. However, alcohol is likely to decrease sexual performance, thus exacerbating the anxiety. In addition, being drunk is fairly unattractive and is likely to put off any potential sexual partner, and so the opportunities for relationships become less. It can be seen from this example that a vicious circle is in force, where sexual anxiety leads to drinking to reduce anxiety, but drinking decreases sexual performance, which leads to more anxiety and the need for greater quantities of alcohol. Upon reading this chapter, it will become apparent that the 'vicious circle' is a common feature in explanations of excessive indulgence.

The costs and benefits of drug use are illustrated in an interesting study by Crawford *et al.* (1983), who interviewed 147 men who had used heroin at some time or other. They classified their sample into four types of user:

1   *light experimenters* (n = 25) who had tried heroin three times or less and then stopped;
2   *moderate experimenters* (n = 17) who had used sporadically, between four and 30 times, and then stopped;
3   *heavy experimenters* (n = 44) who had used regularly, at least 40 times;
4   *addicts* (n = 61) who had used daily for at least three months, experienced withdrawal symptoms, and/or defined themselves as addicts.

They found differences amongst these four groups. Light users did not always get high the first time they tried heroin, and those that did often found the sleepy, sluggish feeling that heroin induces unpleasant. Most preferred some other drug, usually alcohol or marijuana. Fear of addiction, overdosing, or experiencing other adverse consequences were reasons for discontinuing use.

Moderate users had a 'take it or leave it' attitude towards heroin. They were more likely than the light users to enjoy the high, but again they usually preferred alcohol or marijuana. Generally, they snorted the drug rather than injected it. Their drug use was financed mostly through legal means, and they limited their consumption because of the costliness of the drug. They were not heavily involved in a heroin-using subculture.

Careers of heavy users and addicts took similar routes, up to a point. Both groups were heavily involved in other illicit drug use, yet they preferred heroin over other drugs. Their drug use was typically supported by illegal activities, such as drug dealing, shoplifting, burglary and robbery. Heavy users were, however, more likely than addicts to fear addiction and if they experienced withdrawal symptoms they backed off drug use for a while to allow their systems to return to normal. In addition, heavy users continued to associate with non-using friends as well as other heroin users.

Addicts first tried heroin use at a younger age than the others, were more likely to enjoy the high the first time, and were more likely to inject the drug. After the first time, they were more likely purposely to seek out heroin and use it again soon. A significant number of addicts (n = 10) went straight on to daily use. Addicts were less concerned than the others about becoming addicted, although many of them did control their heroin use to a degree, mainly to prevent family and friends finding out that they were using the drug. Many addicts, upon experiencing withdrawal symptoms, used heroin to relieve the unpleasant feelings. This group associated mainly with other users.

Three important factors relating to heavy drug use may be identified in this study:

1   that heavy users claim to experience a strong primary drug reinforcement effect;
2   that heavy users become more involved in a drug subculture; and
3   that heavy users are more likely to take drugs to relieve unpleasant feelings.

These three factors require further exploration.

Drug Reinforcement Effects

Obviously, drugs will affect people differently depending upon their biological make-up. It has already been mentioned in Chapter 2 that Oriental races appear to have a metabolic sensitivity to alcohol that

reduces their likelihood of heavy drinking. Comparison c
with a family history of alcoholism with those with no fam
alcoholism shows that the former are less affected by alcol
this may be based in genetically determined metabolic
(Marshall, 1990). One possible conclusion is that some people may be
disposed to drink more than others because of the comparative lack of
effect alcohol has on them.

Differences may also be found in the neural circuitry of the brain.
Wise (1988) explains the mechanisms of positive and negative reinforcement where drugs are concerned, concluding that these are ana-
tomically and functionally distinct. The positive reinforcing effects of
drugs appear to occur through activation of the dopaminergic system
(dopamine is a neurotransmitter). Negative reinforcing effects, on the
other hand, act through multiple mechanisms involving multiple locations in the brain. Opiates, cocaine, alcohol, nicotine and caffeine activate
the same neural circuitry, which may explain why use of one drug,
such as having a cigarette, can be a risk for relapse to another drug,
such as alcohol.

It seems probable that neural circuitry may differ from one person
to the next, depending upon genetic inheritance, giving rise to variable
sensitivity to positive and negative reinforcement. In support of this,
Cloninger (1987), in a study of adults who were adopted as children,
identified two different types of alcoholism: Type 1 and Type 2. His
Type 1 alcoholics are typified as passive–dependent individuals who
develop alcoholism after the age of 25 years, are binge drinkers, and
rarely get into trouble as a result of their drinking. The genetic background of Type 1 is an alcoholic biological parent, who developed
alcoholism in adulthood and has no history of criminality. Type 2 alcoholics are typically antisocial personalities who develop alcoholism
before they are 25 years old, do not abstain from drinking, and get into
frequent trouble as a result of their drinking. The genetic background
of Type 2 is an alcoholic father, who developed alcoholism early on in
life and who also has a criminal history.

These two types may differ in their neurobiology. Type 1 are low
on novelty-seeking and high on harm avoidance, which suggests that
negative reinforcement systems prevail. Type 2 are high on novelty-
seeking and low on harm avoidance, which suggests that positive reinforcement systems prevail. This may have implications for the potency
or persistence of drug reinforcement; we have already seen that the
typical Type 2 is likely to mature out of drug use, whereas the typical
Type 1 is less likely to do so.

We saw in Chapter 3 that behavioural risk factors for substance use were linked with characteristics such as sensation-seeking and difficult temperament. Temperament issues have been studied from a behavioural–genetic perspective, with some support for hyperactivity and emotionality having a heritable basis (Tarter, 1988). These temperaments are associated with a vulnerability to substance use through interaction with the physical and social environment. For example, a hyperactive child is more likely to get into trouble, fall in with a group of delinquent peers, and use alcohol and drugs because this is the group norm. A person who is emotional may be more vulnerable to using alcohol or drugs to cope with distress.

It is appropriate here to make a statement about the role of genetic research in understanding the observation that addiction runs in families. No genetic marker has been found for alcoholism or drug addiction. The question that must be asked is whether it is reasonable to search for a genetic marker for behaviours as complex as drinking and drug use, bearing in mind all the non-biological factors which influence these behaviours – cultural, social and psychological. There is a qualitative difference here compared to looking for a genetic marker for a biological characteristic, such as gender or eye colour.

Rose *et al.* (1984) argue against 'biological determinism', which holds that

> human lives and actions are inevitable consequences of the biochemical properties of the cells that make up the individual; and these characteristics are in turn uniquely determined by the constituents of the genes possessed by each individual . . . The determinists would have it, then, that human nature is fixed by our genes. (p. 6)

The antithesis to this is the position of 'cultural determinism', where the impact of an individual's biology is considered negligible in comparison with the influences of the culture in which that individual is raised. These opposing positions are, of course, the two poles of the 'nature–nurture' argument.

Few people these days adopt an either/or stance when it comes to the nature–nurture argument; it is obvious that both have a part to play. Individual differences in metabolism, neurobiology and perhaps temperament are likely to be genetically determined and one's inheritance may form a vulnerability factor for the development of addiction. However, a biological predisposition cannot account entirely for a behaviour as complex as substance use; there is an interaction between the person and his or her environment that cannot be ignored.

For example, it is environmental events that activate brain

mechanisms. Reinforcement for drug use and a build up of memories of past reinforcement depend upon an environment which allows drug use to occur. Also, neural circuitry is involved in higher order functioning in terms of reasoning, planning and problem solving; people may be better or worse at these cognitive skills, but so too does the individual's environment affect their development and expression. That is, while biological differences must be taken into account in explaining behaviour, it must not be forgotten that biological, psychological and social factors interact with each other.

Drug Subcultures

Cochrane (1984), in his analysis of the social aspects of drug use, suggests that 'what many addicts are seeking is not the euphoria of heroin intoxication (although they may believe this to be the case) but the socially validated identity of a drug addict' (p. 132). When a person begins to use drugs, it is often the case that the physical experience is either minimal or unpleasant. For continuation of drug use, that person must be prepared to learn how to respond, and one of the motivating forces for bothering to learn is to fit in with the drug using subculture. It may be that within this subculture, the 'addict' finds a socially validated role that allows for the possibilities of success and status, in much the same way as for those who adopt a conventional role in society.

Cochrane goes on to draw similarities between work and heroin addiction. Work imposes a structure on the day, and compels one to be active; heroin addiction requires a person to make efforts to obtain supplies. Work requires that people come into contact with each other and collaborate to attain goals; heroin addiction demands that connections be made with drug dealers and that each party trusts the other to avoid contact with the law. Work confers status and identity through being something – a mechanic, a nurse, a teacher or whatever – and this identity is reflected in the language, skills and customs of that group; heroin addiction confers a similar group status and identity, with its own language (the impenetrable drug jargon), skills (e.g. the ability to manage overdoses), and customs (e.g. the rituals surrounding drug-taking).

Involvement in the drug using subculture can be amplified by social labelling effects. The public holds a stereotype of drug users as immoral, lazy and criminal. The police are motivated by public pressure to act against drug users, and the drug using group has to adapt to this situation. They, therefore, become more segregated from society and more cohesive as a group. The stereotype becomes a self-fulfilling prophecy and public censure becomes even greater. Caught in this vicious circle, the drug user finds it increasingly difficult to abandon this way of life and return to 'normal' society (see Cochrane, 1984).

Support for the notion of 'addiction to being an addict', comes from a study of Canadian heroin addicts in Britain (Zacune, 1976). In the 1960s, because maintenance prescription was legal in the UK but not in Canada, a number of Canadian addicts migrated to Britain. Their reasons for leaving Canada were so that they could avoid drug-related crime, and hence avoid jail, and so that they could lead normal lives. A follow-up of the 91 émigrés showed that 10 had died in Britain, and 10 had been deported. Of the remaining 71, it is interesting to note that about half (35) had returned to Canada voluntarily because they were missing the 'street life' that is part of the drug scene. Interviews with 25 of those remaining in Britain, after they had been in Britain for almost six years, showed that most (but not all) were indeed leading 'normal' lives, that is they were working and staying out of trouble with the law.

This study shows that some people are indeed 'addicted to being an addict' and cannot live apart from the drug scene; others, however, make a decision to change and to effect this change it is helpful to extricate themselves from the drug scene. Indeed, we saw in the last chapter that factors involved in giving up drug use are those related to work, marriage and family. That is, the user retires from the drug using subculture to adopt a more conventional role in society.

Relief of Unpleasant Feelings

The belief that addiction to a substance or activity is maintained by warding off unpleasant feelings is widely held. Unpleasant feelings include both physical distress and psychological distress.

Coping with Physical Distress

It is important at the outset to make two points clear. The first is that it is incontrovertible that some people experience adverse physical effects when they are deprived of a drug that they have been taking regularly. The second point is that while these withdrawal effects may have a biological basis in part, psychological factors also have a role to play. These claims require further elucidation.

When a person uses a drug repeatedly, the effectiveness of that drug diminishes, that is *tolerance* develops. The development of tolerance means that larger amounts of the drug need to be taken to produce the same effects that were previously acquired with smaller doses. The presence of tolerance is usually accompanied by evidence of *withdrawal* symptoms, that is the adverse physical effects that are experienced when the person is deprived of the drug.

Tolerance and withdrawal undoubtedly have a biological basis. Biological explanations of drug tolerance include changes in drug metabolism, where the drug is broken down more rapidly and so less is available for pharmacological activity (dispositional tolerance), and neuroadaptation, where neural adjustments take place to counteract the acute effects of the drug (functional tolerance). In each case, more and more of the drug becomes necessary to have an effect. Where neuroadaptation has occurred, changes in the synthesis, storage, or release of neurotransmitters, or changes in receptor sensitivity, may produce withdrawal symptoms in the absence of the drug (Madden, 1984).

Withdrawal symptoms vary across drugs. Alcohol withdrawal symptoms include tremor, sweating, nausea and vomiting. The most severe form of withdrawal symptom is delirium tremens, commonly known as 'the DTs'. Here, the whole body shakes, consciousness is clouded and hallucinations may be experienced. Hallucinations are often very frightening, such as seeing mice, spiders or snakes (perhaps even pink elephants) in the room. Opioid withdrawal features include anxiety, restlessness, yawning, running nose, watering eyes, aching muscles, stomach cramps, nausea, vomiting and diarrhoea (Madden, 1984). Some drugs, such as amphetamines, LSD and cannabis cause little in the way of withdrawal symptoms.

It seems reasonable to suppose that drinking or drug use will occur to relieve these unpleasant symptoms. However, as Orford (1985) points out, the act of drug-taking to relieve withdrawal symptoms is *learned*. The knowledge that taking the 'hair of the dog that bit you' is passed on in drinking and drug-using lore, and trying this cure is reinforced through processes of operant conditioning. In addition to this, it will become apparent in the next section when cue reactivity is discussed, that both tolerance and withdrawal may be *classically conditioned responses*. That is, some of the physical effects of drugs can be accounted for by psychological processes.

To conclude this section, it is important to highlight the vicious circle that arises with the use of drugs to relieve withdrawal symptoms. Orford (1985) says that 'If the sequence of withdrawing, experiencing stressful withdrawal symptoms, taking a further dose, and experiencing relief of withdrawal, is followed repeatedly, the motivation to consume the drug regularly will be much increased' (p. 194).

Coping with Psychological Distress

The belief that drugs and alcohol are sometimes used in coping with unpleasant emotions lies behind clichés such as 'drinking your troubles away' and using drugs to 'escape from reality'. The hypothesis that alcohol reduces tension, anxiety or stress (these three terms being broadly synonymous) has been investigated over many years. In his review of the literature on alcohol and anxiety, Wilson (1988) points out that there have been conflicting findings regarding alcohol's effects; alcohol has been variously shown to decrease anxiety, increase it, or have no effect on it. Some of this inconsistency may be explained in methodological terms, for example that researchers have used different definitions and measures of anxiety, yet there is more to it than this. The question 'Does alcohol reduce anxiety?' is conceptually naive, and a better question to ask is 'At what dose, under which conditions, in whom, and on what measures does alcohol reduce anxiety?' (Wilson, 1988). One important development in this field of study is the incorporation of outcome expectancies into the equation. Expectancies may be one mediating factor in stress reduction – those who expect alcohol (or other drugs) to transform negative moods into positive ones may be more likely to drink heavily.

Cooper *et al.* (1988) studied drinking to cope, which they define as 'the tendency to use alcohol to escape, avoid or otherwise regulate unpleasant emotions' (p. 218). Along with measures of drinking to cope, they measured alcohol-related outcome expectancies, presuming that the belief that alcohol will ameliorate unpleasant emotions would be necessary for a person to use alcohol for coping purposes. In a comparison of alcohol abusers and non-abusers, they found that

> individuals who hold strong positive expectancies and also use avoidant styles of coping with emotion were most likely to drink to cope. In turn, individuals who hold strong positive expectancies and who drink to cope not only drink more, but are also more likely to experience problems as a result of their drinking. (Cooper *et al.*, 1988, p. 228)

These findings suggest that some people have difficulty managing their emotions and, if they expect alcohol to help them cope, then they are at risk of becoming heavy drinkers. They differ from social drinkers, who hold positive alcohol-related outcome expectancies, but do not use alcohol for coping with their emotions, perhaps because they possess other coping skills. Those who drink to cope are more likely to experience alcohol-related problems, suggesting that drinking to cope may be intrinsically maladaptive. That is, there exists the opportunity for a vicious circle to develop. An example of this was given earlier where the person drank to cope with feelings of sexual inadequacy; although drinking may initially help alleviate anxiety, alcohol actually decreases sexual performance, thus creating the conditions for increased anxiety, and, paradoxically, even greater levels of drinking.

Gender differences are apparent in alcohol outcome expectancies. One interesting finding in relation to tension reduction is that while women hold the belief that alcohol reduces tension, in social situations the actual effect of alcohol consumption is to *increase* tension. The tension reduction expectancy may need to be balanced against other expectancies, in this case that alcohol leads to cognitive and physical impairment (Young *et al.*, 1990). It is reasonable to suppose that some women will not be prepared to risk drinking heavily in social situations, since the cognitive and physical impairment that results may make them feel vulnerable to undesirable events.

One frequently cited difference between male and female 'alcoholics' is that women are more likely to experience emotional problems, and more often attribute their drinking to stress (Lex, 1991). Female 'alcoholics' are more likely to feel guilty, anxious or depressed, but then women do experience more social disapproval for alcohol use, to the degree of stigmatization where drinking is excessive. It is hard to tease out cause and effect; do women drink to cope with psychological distress, or does social ostracism consequent upon women's drinking cause psychological distress? Another vicious circle bares its teeth.

One proposed mechanism whereby alcohol effects tension reduction is that it narrows attention. Josephs and Steele (1990) call this 'alcohol myopia'. What happens is that alcohol reduces one's attentional capacity such that the demands of ongoing activity take up all one's attention, leaving no room for attention to stressful thoughts, and so anxiety is reduced. Josephs and Steele (1990) investigated this experimentally. Their subjects were given a drink; half of the subjects were given alcohol and the other half were given no alcohol, although all were told that the drinks contained alcohol. Anxiety was raised by telling the subjects that they would be required to give a speech on the topic of 'What I dislike about my body and my physical appearance'. Anxiety levels were measured at this point.

Subjects were then split into two groups. The first group was asked to sit quietly and do nothing; the second group was occupied by being asked to rate a series of art slides. Attention was therefore taken up by alcohol, which reduces attentional capacity, and/or the task, which requires concentration. The hypothesis was that all subjects in the group engaged in the rating task would show reduced anxiety because their attention was taken up with the task, and that this effect would be greater for those who had drunk alcohol. Where subjects were doing nothing, they expected all subjects to show an increase in anxiety, but that those who had drunk alcohol would show a greater increase than subjects who had not drunk alcohol. Because attentional capacity is limited by drinking, there will be a tendency for the drinkers to focus on what is going on in the present, in this case the prospect of making an embarrassing speech. Those who had not drunk any alcohol would have a wider attention capacity and would therefore be able to think about coping strategies.

These hypotheses were broadly supported in the study, allowing the conclusion that alcohol reduces attentional capacity such that the drinker focuses his or her attention upon immediate concerns and has no spare capacity for attention to stressful thoughts. Of course, distraction works for sober people as well, but where drink is involved less demanding activities are required to take one's mind off one's worries. Josephs and Steele point out that it seldom happens in the real world that people drink and do absolutely nothing else. Most drinkers are engaged in some activity – whether chatting with friends, watching television, or reading the paper. These activities suffice to take up the attention of the 'alcohol myopic' such that drinking reliably reduces tension.

To summarize, excessive indulgence in an addictive behaviour may be understood using the same principles as for moderate indulgence. People drink heavily or use drugs excessively because of the overall reinforcement for doing so. Negative reinforcement has a large part to play in that the 'addict' often engages in the addictive behaviour to avoid or relieve unpleasant states, particularly physical and emotional discomfort. The phenomenon of diminished control must now be addressed.

Diminished Control

Heather (1991), in his analysis of impaired control over alcohol consumption, makes a number of important points. First, he asks what is meant by impaired control. Researchers have investigated a diverse range of phenomena, including inability to stop, inability to abstain, trying to stop or cut down but failing, getting drunk at inappropriate times or places, drinking alone and worrying about drinking. Clearly, impaired control means different things to different people. This indicates the need for an agreed definition of loss of control for use in research. Heather suggests quite simply that loss of control may be defined as the likelihood of continued drinking after a given amount of alcohol.

Heather goes on to point out that it is necessary also to take into account the drinker's intention. Control is not an issue for many 'alcoholics'. While some are able to control their drinking should they wish to do so (as we have seen in Chapter 1), the notion of control is irrelevant to many others; they have no wish to control their drinking and never attempt to exercise control. What we must look at, then, is impaired control over drinking and other drug use given the intention of exercising control.

What factors, then, may be implicated in the likelihood of continued drinking and drug use despite the person's intention to remain abstinent or moderate? The issues to be covered in this section include strong desire, cognitive functioning and self-efficacy.

Strong Desire

The expression of 'craving' is a phenomenon that cannot be ignored when it comes to the study of those who are heavily involved in an addictive behaviour. Many theorists hold that craving captures the essence of addiction, yet there is much controversy about what the term actually means. Kozlowski and Wilkinson (1987) point out that craving is a word in common usage that has been adopted by scientists and put into technical service, without having an agreed definition. In the vernacular, craving means a strong desire or intense longing, and its use in relation to addictive behaviours imputes an unnecessary degree of intensity to the feeling. If one were to talk about desires or urges, with craving being reserved for the strongest urges, then the phenomenon would be put into perspective. Despite advice from experts to abandon the term craving, researchers have shown remarkable persistence in its use. However, the term adopted in this chapter is 'desire'.

As it is, desire is understood in various ways by its investigators. Some hold that it has a physiological basis, such as an underlying tissue-need for a drug, and others construe desire as a psychological phenomenon. These two conceptualizations lead to the differentiation between *physical dependence* and *psychological dependence*. Attempts have been made to separate these two aspects of desire, but this has generally served to obscure rather than clarify the issue. The reason for this is that there is an interrelationship between physical and psychological elements, and both must be taken into account in explaining desire – of any magnitude – to engage in an addictive behaviour. One particularly useful direction in this research area has been the study of cue reactivity.

It has been observed that cues associated with substance use can elicit various conditioned responses, a phenomenon called *cue reactivity*. An example is an experiment by Pomerleau *et al.* (1983), who compared cue reactivity in male alcohol abusers and male moderate drinkers. Their subjects were told that the experiment concerned an assessment of the pleasantness of different substances and they were asked to sniff cedar chips or a favourite alcoholic beverage. The experimenters took various measures before and after sniffing, including swallowing, ratings of desire to drink, and physiological measures, such as heart rate and skin conductance. Their results showed that alcohol abusers were more reactive to alcohol-related stimuli than were people with a history of moderation, and that swallowing (i.e. salivation) and expressed desire to drink were the two measures which best differentiated the abusers from the non-abusers.

In their review of cue reactivity in the addictive behaviours, Rohsenow *et al.* (1991) provide evidence for a similar reactivity to physical cues for smokers, heroin users and cocaine users. Exposure to cigarettes, lighters, ashtrays and the like increases urges to smoke, speeds up smoking and raises blood pressure. Tapes of drug talk, pictures of drug paraphernalia and videotapes of drug administration rituals result in increased desire for drugs, and changes in physiological measures, such as respiration and temperature, in both heroin and cocaine addicts. Rohsenow *et al.* (1991) point out that it is not only physical cues which elicit this reactivity, but also internal cues such as states resembling withdrawal, negative emotional states and positive emotional states. In fact, the cues that precipitate drinking and drug use may be highly complex. The sight of the hardware, such as bottles, needles and so on, may not have much of an impact compared with the cue complex of setting, plus companions, plus time, plus mood. Compare, for example, the likely strength of desire to drink of a young man in a city centre pub on Saturday night, with heavy drinking friends who are looking for fun, as opposed to the same young man in a country pub on a Sunday afternoon, with his parents having a drink before lunch.

One cue which deserves a specific mention is that of a *priming dose*, which has been researched in the alcohol field. Experimental findings in this area have been summarized by Stockwell (1991). After imbibing a quantity of alcohol (a priming dose), the desire to drink is increased, with priming effects being most evident under the following conditions:

1   where the setting is highly similar to the real-life drinking setting;
2   with higher priming doses of alcohol;
3   when the subject's preferred alcoholic beverage was used for the priming dose;
4   when further alcoholic drinks are available for consumption, and the drinker knows this to be so; and
5   when subjects are severely dependent upon alcohol, or, put another way, when subjects have long reinforcement histories for heavy alcohol use.

The observation that exposure to cues related to alcohol or a drug elicits a desire to indulge in that substance raises the important question of whether this desire actually predicts behaviour. Desire may be seen as a precursor to loss of control in that a preoccupation with thinking about the object of desire may lead to actions directed at fulfilling that desire. Desire may be a useful construct only if it predicts drinking or drug use; that is, the experience of desire might not be of particular concern to anyone if it simply existed on its own without being translated into action.

Rankin *et al.* (1979) attempted to measure a behavioural correlate of 'craving' in alcoholics. Ten subjects were recruited and their feelings of craving were experimentally manipulated. All were allowed to drink 'as normal' before the experiment started, and thereafter half were asked to refrain from drinking (high craving), while the other half were allowed to continue drinking up to the behavioural test (low craving). The behavioural test was to provide each subject with two glasses of vodka and tonic to drink in their own time. Subjects in the high craving condition drank faster, and the greater their reported level of desire, the faster the drinking speed.

Marlatt (1985a), in an analysis of situations that precipitated relapse to a number of problem behaviours (drinking, smoking, heroin use, gambling and overeating), found that urges and temptations did account for a proportion of relapses, although the front runner by far was negative emotional states. Of course, as Heather and Stallard (1989) point out, relapse was assigned to the 'urges and temptations' category only where no other category of interpersonal or intrapersonal factors applied. They go on to say that there are usually multiple reasons for relapse, and that craving may be one of these, but only identified as such under some circumstances. They provide the example of a smoker who has given up for a few weeks and is still feeling the desire for a cigarette. After an argument at home, he storms out of the house and goes to the pub. Here he meets an old friend – a heavy smoker – who urges him to have a cigarette. After a few drinks, he gives in and lights up. If the smoker were asked 'What caused the relapse?', he would be unable to give one single reason. The desire for a cigarette played its part in this tale, but equally the relapse could be attributed to the argument with the wife, the social pressure of the old friend, or the consumption of alcohol. He might be least likely to give desire as the primary reason for giving in.

Heather and Stallard (1989) show that the way the research question is asked can make more or less of the impact played by desire. In their study, when heroin users were asked specifically about desire as a reason for relapse, many more cited this as relevant than in Marlatt's study. Another factor is time since giving up. In a study of smokers, Velicer *et al.* (1990) found that 'cravings' accounted for relapse much more in the early stages of giving up; in the later stages, relapse was attributed more to negative emotional states.

It seems fair to conclude that exposure to cues related to the addictive behaviour elicits a desire to indulge, and that, in turn, this desire predicts actual behaviour. Of course, this is not to say that desire *always* leads to drinking or drug use; it is obviously possible for some people to resist temptation. This suggests that other factors play their part, for example weighing up the advantages of giving up versus giving in.

One important point, however, is the wide range of cues that can come to elicit reactivity. Gossop (1990) provides a list of cues that have regularly been found to elicit desire in heroin addicts. These are presented in Table 4.2. What becomes clear is that the cues that precipitate desire in heavy users are numerous and diverse. Many sights, thoughts and feelings trigger off the desire to use. It would seem impossible to avoid many of these cues, therefore it is important that we should strive to understand cue reactivity and its clinical implications.

Table 4.2   *Cues which elicit craving (Gossop, 1990)*

Seeing someone you know who is a heroin user
Being in a place associated in some way with opiates
Seeing needles or syringes
Seeing silver foil
Passing a chemist
When you are feeling bored
Being in a pub
Having a single drink of alcohol
When you are feeling angry, worried or anxious
Using a drug like cannabis
Thinking about yourself using opiates
Thinking about people you know who use opiates
Using a drug like cocaine

Cue reactivity may be explained in a number of ways. In classical conditioning terms, drug administration (unconditioned stimulus) leads to the drug effects (unconditioned response). Drug administration is paired with drug-related cues (conditioned stimuli) that acquire the power to elicit the conditioned response. There is some controversy about the nature of the conditioned response, which differs depending upon the model one follows. Some theorists say that conditioned stimuli elicit a state similar to the drug effect, and that this stimulates an urge to use the drug. Others say that the unconditioned response is in the opposite direction to the drug effect (e.g. opponent process theory), leading to withdrawal distress and to the desire to use the drug to relieve this unpleasant state.

In operant terms, cues operate as discriminative stimuli, signalling the possibility of reward for drinking or drug use. Over time, many discriminative stimuli acquire power to elicit the addictive behaviour, and so the behaviour generalizes to a wide range of stimuli or settings. This occurs when the incentives are strong and the disincentives relatively weak, such that discrimination is eroded (Orford, 1985).

Hodgson (1990) explains that desire does not occur in a vacuum, but that it is linked to the antecedents and consequences of a behaviour and, just as importantly, to the person's outcome expectancies. He suggests that a strong desire is based upon the expected positive outcomes of a behaviour, and the expected negative outcomes of not engaging in that behaviour. For example, a strong desire to visit the pub the morning after the night before may be based upon 'a desire to reduce the shakes, keep withdrawal symptoms at bay, enjoy the social stimulation, possibly experience euphoria, blot out family problems, reduce anxiety, and avoid the frustration which would occur if drinking

Table 4.3   *Capabilities required for self-control (after Wilkinson, 1991)*

1   Planning ability
2   Restraint and inhibition
3   Cognitive adaptability
4   Ability to modulate arousal
5   Persistence with goal-directed strategies

was resisted' (Hodgson, 1990, p. 229). The heart of desire, he says, is the anticipation of pleasure and/or pleasurable relief.

Cognitive Functioning

As we have already seen, there may be genetically determined differences in the neural circuitry of the brain. These may influence drug reinforcement properties, but they may also affect cognitive functioning. Parsons (1989) studied Type 1 and Type 2 alcoholics on a variety of neuropsychological tests. He found that Type 1 males scored lower than Type 2 males on tests of learning, memory, problem-solving and perceptual-motor tasks, and that Type 1 males performed less well where a family history of alcoholism was evident, compared to those Type 1s where there was no family history. These results suggest that male Type 1 alcoholics, especially if they have a family history of alcoholism, are likely to show marked neuropsychological deficits.

While deficits in cognitive functioning may be inherited by individuals, it is also true to say that drug use may cause damage to the central nervous system. This is certainly evident where alcohol use is concerned. Wilkinson (1991) in his review of the effects of alcohol on the brain concludes that 'alcohol dependent patients with long histories of dependence tend to have marked abnormalities of cerebral morphology that suggest diffuse brain injury with particular vulnerability of the frontal cortex' (p. 115). To understand this, we need to know the role of the frontal lobes in the control of behaviour. Wilkinson points out that the frontal lobes are responsible for the very capabilities required for self-control, which are summarized in Table 4.3. Wilkinson suggests, therefore, that impaired control may be a neuropsychological consequence of alcohol dependence. He goes on to suggest that such brain injury would impair control in other areas besides drinking; that is the person would have difficulty controlling not only his or her drinking, but other behaviours as well. This may go some way to explaining the relationship between heavy drinking and behaviours such as violence and sexual disinhibition.

Coping Skills and Self-efficacy

The use of alcohol and drugs for coping with emotional distress was discussed earlier in this chapter. When people decide to stop or cut down their drinking or drug use, two major issues relating to coping arise. First, the change in substance use itself creates specific problems, such as the need to resist the desire to drink or use drugs. Second, in the absence of substance use, the problems for which drinking and drug use were previously used as a palliative become evident. The individual may not possess the skills required for dealing with these problems, in which case a relapse to substance use as a means of coping is likely. Alternatively, the individual may know what action is required to solve the problem, but simply not have sufficient confidence in his or her abilities to make an active attempt at problem solving; again, relapse to substance use is likely.

Clearly, individuals vary in their problem solving abilities, depending partly on natural talents and partly on learning history. While impaired cognitive abilities, as mentioned above, may affect problem solving ability, factors relating to motivation to engage in problem solving are also important. Cynn (1992) assessed motivation to engage in problem-solving tasks (tracing geometric diagrams without lifting the pencil, solving anagrams and sorting cards) by measuring how long alcohol-dependent and non-dependent control subjects persisted at these tasks. She found that her alcohol-dependent subjects gave up sooner than her controls, but that their problem-solving abilities were intact. Her subjects were young (early thirties) and healthy, and it may be that cognitive impairment becomes more evident with increasing age and duration of alcohol dependence. Nevertheless, it is clear that motivation plays an important role in problem-solving abilities.

Self-efficacy (see the section on social learning theory in Chapter 2) has been defined as the person's evaluation of his or her competence to perform a task in a given situation. The level of confidence a person has in his or her ability to cope successfully will determine the selection of coping behaviours and the degree of persistence in their execution. An example of this might be a woman who drinks at home alone because she is lonely. This woman may be quite aware of the fact that drinking is merely a palliative, and that the best solution in the long term would be to take up activities that would create opportunities to meet people and make friends. She may have ideas about various activities that might be appropriate: joining a social club, going to classes, or taking up a sport. What may prevent her actually doing any of these is the belief that even if she were introduced to new people, her social skills would let her down; she would be unable to start or sustain a conversation, or she would say or do the wrong thing. Rather than risk appearing dull or making a social gaffe, it is easier to stay home and find a friend in alcohol.

Integration

The purpose of this chapter was to explain dependence, and a summary and integration of the information presented is required for clarity's sake.

First of all, a person engaging in an addictive behaviour does so because the overall *balance of costs and benefits favours a positive outcome*. Social, psychological and biological factors all influence the costs and benefits present in the individual's balance, and so each individual has a unique degree of vulnerability to indulgence in any addictive behaviour.

The addictive behaviour is reinforced in a variety of ways for each individual, including social validation and relief of unpleasant feelings. Reasons and rewards for the behaviour are often reciprocally bound in a *vicious circle*, such that the level of the behaviour increases. That is, the rewards contingent upon the addictive behaviour are readily accessible and these are sought for short term gain, yet in the longer term the addictive behaviour exacerbates or creates problems, leading to an increase in the addictive behaviour.

Diminished control over the behaviour becomes evident when attempts are made to stop or cut down. The concept of control makes little sense in the absence of a change attempt. The factors contributing to the experience of diminished control may best be described within the framework of *self-regulation*, which has its basis in conditioning and social learning theories (see Chapter 2). The process of self-regulation consists of several components, including receiving and processing information about one's behaviour, making decisions about change, planning for change, successfully executing an action plan, and evaluating the outcome. These processes may be disrupted in various ways, leading to the experience of diminished control.

The person must first of all be aware of his or her behaviour, the environmental factors that trigger that behaviour, and the consequences which maintain it. As we have seen, *cue reactivity* to stimuli associated with the addictive behaviour develops as a consequence of many behavioural events (e.g. drinking or drug use) occurring in the presence of those cues. The number and range of cues becomes ever wider, such that many settings, situations and feelings trigger off the desire to indulge in the addictive behaviour. This phenomenon is usually *beyond the conscious information processing* of the individual concerned. Attempts to change are thwarted by these unrecognized obstacles, and so the behaviour seems to be out of personal control.

Some people, notably drinkers, may have suffered *cognitive impairment* as a consequence of their behaviour. Where once the individual could easily exercise the cognitive skills necessary for self-regulation, this may have become more of a challenge. While decisions to change may be made, cognitive impairment militates against the formulation of effective action plans, and so *action plans are inadequate* to carry out those decisions. The experience here is of loss of an ability to exercise control where once there existed that ability.

Where the addictive behaviour has been used as a means of coping with life's problems, stopping or reducing the addictive behaviour can serve to make those *problems more salient*. In addition, *fresh problems may arise*, such as the need for skills to cope with the desire to indulge which is elicited by abstention. These problems may overwhelm the person who is trying to make changes. Where skills are lacking, the easiest route is to return to the addictive behaviour as a coping strategy, thus giving the sense of being out of control.

These failures of self-regulation result in *lowered self-efficacy expectations*, that is, the person begins to believe that he or she cannot exercise the necessary control, leading to the belief that one cannot change. In conjunction with this, *positive outcome expectancies are maintained* in relation to the addictive behaviour, increasing the likelihood of increased indulgence.

The typical outcome with those who experience failures in self-regulation is the employment of defensive tactics, rather than change strategies, to reduce the discrepancy between actual behaviour and the internal standard. These may include reappraisal of the information ('I don't drink as much as some people do'), modification of the decision to change ('I didn't want to stop anyway'), or reassessment of the options ('It's not my problem; if they are bothered by it, let them change').

These defensive strategies are commonly labelled *denial,* that is the 'addict' is viewed as being blind to the fact that he or she has a problem.

The implications contained in the integration statement above are that change may be assisted in a number of ways. One option is to introduce the person engaged in the addictive behaviour to alternative sources of reinforcement, for example through occupational, social and leisure activities. Control clearly must be re-established, and training in techniques of self-regulation are important. Coping skills for maintenance of change are obviously required, and help may be given through training in techniques for assertiveness, social skills, and tension reduction. Change is the topic of the next chapter, where these and other interventions will be described.

Chapter 5

Change

Many therapeutic interventions have been developed to help people with addictions. These include a range of therapies based upon psychological principles, as well as detoxification, drug treatments, rehabilitation, twelve-step programmes (e.g. Alcoholics Anonymous, Narcotics Anonymous, Gamblers Anonymous) and therapeutic communities. Because this book is about the psychology of addiction, psychological interventions will be most fully described in this chapter, however, other approaches commonly used in practice will also be mentioned, albeit briefly. In looking at the application of cognitive-behavioural interventions with addictive behaviours, it has been noted in a recent review that there is a 'disappointing lack of attention being paid to drug classes other than alcohol' (Mattick and Heather, 1993, p. 424). Evidence for the effectiveness of these interventions with both alcohol and drug users is presented where possible, however, in some cases evaluated interventions with drinkers may be the only evidence available.

In general, levels of success in intervention are modest. Orford's (1985) overall conclusion, after reading reports of the effectiveness of programmes for obesity, excessive drinking, and excessive drug use, is that at follow-up 6–12 months after the intervention, on average one-third of clients have improved. On the basis of this, some critics would hold that interventions for addictions are not particularly effective; after all two-thirds of clients either do not improve at all or improve only temporarily, soon slipping back into their old habits. In response to this challenge, it could be said that only the most difficult cases ask for formal help, and that the success rate is therefore more impressive than it seems to be at first sight. Of course, the statement that only difficult cases ask for help implies that some people can change addictive behaviours on their own. This is indeed so; many people do change without professional help. Before going on to describe interventions, we shall take a look at this group of people who change without assistance to glean clues about how interventions might best be designed.

Advances in knowledge about the development of addiction and processes of change has altered therapists' views of how best to organize services for clients. Instead of promoting this or that brand of therapy as the best in the field, there is a growing awareness that different clients require different interventions at different stages in the process of change. Matching the client with the intervention is a considerably more sophisticated approach than offering all comers the same package, and holds promise for improving therapeutic outcomes. Issues relating to matching will be presented here.

First, a word about terminology is necessary. In this chapter, 'intervention' is used as a generic term to describe any procedure a professional may use to help a client change. Use of the word 'treatment' has been avoided because of its medical connotations; the person who seeks help with an addiction problem is not ill. 'Treatment' also implies the administration of a procedure selected by an 'expert' and delivered to a passive recipient. In psychological therapies, the client is informed about alternative goals and the range of methods for achieving these goals, so that he or she may choose from the options available. This process of negotiation is likely to enhance the client's commitment to any change programme.

Unassisted Change

In the field of addictions, it has been observed that large numbers of people successfully change their behaviour from uncontrolled use to moderation or abstinence without receiving any help. Unassisted change has been termed 'maturing out' or 'spontaneous remission'. Implicit in the term 'maturing out' is the notion that heavy drinkers or drug users are somehow 'immature' and that the passage of time leads to greater 'maturity' and therefore to controlled use (Yates, 1990). The term 'spontaneous remission' is clearly based on the medical model, and implicit here is the notion that change is in the nature of a miracle cure. Neither of these terms is satisfactory, since they stand in the way of any investigation of the factors that enable people to regain control of their behaviour. It is not the passage of time in itself that accounts for change, but what happens during that time (Yates, 1990). It is only relatively recently that investigators have made attempts to study the reasons for and processes of self-change. One purpose behind such research is to gather information which may be of use in clinical practice; since more people give up or cut down by their own efforts than through professional help, there may be important lessons to be learned from this group.

Tuchfeld (1981) studied 51 men and women who reported having had alcohol problems that they resolved without recourse to formal intervention, 40 becoming abstinent and 11 drinking moderately. Many of these subjects had rejected the possibility of formal treatment because they did not wish to be labelled 'alcoholic'. As one interviewee put it, 'Would you want somebody to call you "cancerous" if you had cancer?' (Tuchfeld, 1981, p. 630). Their reasons for initiating change were experiencing an illness or having an accident; extraordinary events, such as a humiliating experience, a suicide attempt, or seeing other heavy drinkers and thinking 'That could be me'; religious conversion; financial problems; direct intervention by family or friends; alcohol-related death or illness of another person; education about 'alcoholism'; and alcohol-related legal problems. Tuchfeld noticed that the resolution of alcohol problems involved a process of change, including a recognition of the problem, disengagement from alcohol-related social and leisure activities, and modification of self-concept towards seeing oneself as a worthwhile and competent person.

Self-change has been further analysed by Stall and Biernacki (1986), who looked at factors important to ending problematic substance use in the literature about alcohol, opiates, tobacco and food/obesity. They identified a number of common factors from which they derived a model of 'spontaneous remission' behaviour. This model consists of three stages of change:

1 *motivation*, where the negative consequences of substance use, such as health problems, social sanctions, interpersonal problems and financial difficulties lead to a decision to quit misuse;
2 *action*, where the remitter makes a public statement of intention to change, thereby committing himself or herself to taking the steps necessary for stopping or cutting down; and
3 *management*, where the remitter creates a new non-using identity, by changing his or her lifestyle to enable change to be maintained.

These studies of unassisted change suggest first that it may be counterproductive to attempt to label a person an 'alcoholic' or an 'addict' in the attempt to engage that person in a therapeutic intervention. Second, decision-making, action and management may be issues that must be dealt with in that order. It makes sense to suppose that change efforts should be based upon a firm commitment to change before they can be applied effectively. This idea of change as a *process* rather than an event has been developed for clinical practice in the stages of change model, which will be described next.

Stages of Change

Prochaska *et al.* (1992) describe a comprehensive model of change in addictive behaviours. They have identified five well-defined stages which form a predictable motivational route from the position of not recognizing a problem, through recognition and change, to the point at which the problem no longer exists. These five stages are as follows:

1 *Precontemplation* is where the person is unaware of or not particularly concerned by the consequences of his or her behaviour, and there is no intention to change in the foreseeable future. An example here might be the smoker who says 'I know smoking is harmful, but I've been smoking since I was 17 years old and I'm not going to stop now.'

2 *Contemplation* is where the person is aware that a problem exists, and is seriously contemplating change, yet there is no firm commitment to take action. Here, the smoker might say 'Smoking is a bad habit and I must do something about it, but I get so irritable when I can't have a cigarette that stopping means I've got to risk falling out with people.'

3 *Preparation* is where the person has decided to change in the near future. A good example here is the New Year's resolution. The smoker may decide to give up on 1 January, and may make preparations to do so by advising friends not to give him or her cigarettes as a Christmas gift.

4 *Action* is where the person effects change. The smoker may dispose of cigarettes, lighters and ashtrays; buy nicotine replacement chewing gum or patches; and refuse offers of cigarettes with the announcement 'I've stopped smoking'.

5 *Maintenance* is where the person consolidates the behaviour change over time. The former smoker will begin to change his or her self-image from smoker to non-smoker. Taking up a sport, for example, helps keep one's weight in check and contributes to a self-image of being fit and healthy, which is incompatible with the self-image of being a smoker.

While some people may progress smoothly from precontemplation through contemplation, preparation and action to maintenance, most people *relapse*. That is, it is rare to succeed in the first attempt to change, and many revert to their previous behaviour pattern at some point. Relapsers regress to an earlier stage in the model, for example from action back to contemplation or preparation. Some people may relapse and recycle through the stages several times, however, the process of taking action and relapsing allows people to learn from experience, and they may be better equipped to succeed in their next change attempt. Others may get stuck in one or other of the stages for a long time. The 'chronic contemplator' is one example, typified by the person who says he or she is going to quit smoking, cut down drinking, or go on a diet, but always starting tomorrow.

One implication of the stages of change model is that people may require different kinds of intervention depending upon which stage they are at when help is sought. It may be fruitless, for example, to direct someone into an action-oriented programme when they are in the contemplation stage. This is the concept of matching clients with interventions.

Matching Clients with Interventions

Any search for a single, universally successful intervention for addictive behaviours may be likened to a search for a unicorn. The question to ask is not 'What works?', but rather 'What interventions work best with which clients?' This question captures the essence of the *matching hypothesis*, whose three key principles are outlined by Miller and Hester (1989, p. 11):

1 There is no single superior approach to treatment for all individuals.
2 Different individuals respond best to different treatment approaches.
3 It is possible to match individuals to optimal treatments, thereby increasing treatment effectiveness and efficiency.

The issue that arises from the matching hypothesis is to establish on what basis decisions may be made about what intervention might be best for whom.

Table 5.1 *Therapist's tasks (after Miller and Rollnick, 1991)*

Client stage	Therapist's tasks
Precontemplation	Increase the client's perception of risks and problems with current behaviour.
Contemplation	Evoke reasons to change and increase client's self-efficacy for change.
Preparation	Help the client determine the best course of action.
Action	Help the client take steps towards change.
Maintenance	Help the client prevent relapse.
Relapse	Help the client to renew the processes of contemplation, preparation and action.

The stages of change model provides some information about what types of intervention may be appropriate for people in any stage. Studies of how people move from one stage to the next have provided information about *processes of change*, such as consciousness raising (i.e. gathering information about the problem), self-evaluation (i.e. assessing how one feels and thinks about oneself with regard to the problem), and self-liberation (i.e. making a commitment to change). Different processes are relevant at different stages of change. Precontemplators are not given to examining themselves or their problems, and are not active in making change attempts. Contemplators are open to information and self-evaluation. Those in the preparation stage continue with self-evaluation, and may be taking initial steps towards action. During the action stage, techniques to control behaviour are used increasingly, and there is reliance on helping relationships. In maintenance, alternative coping responses are developed. Knowledge about these processes and their application at different stages of change provide guidance regarding the therapist's task at each stage. These tasks have been defined by Miller and Rollnick (1991) as shown in Table 5.1.

These tasks may be broadly grouped into five intervention modules, as shown in Figure 5.1 (McMurran and Hollin, 1993). These modules each contain a number of approaches, gathered together to make some effort to indicate how clients may be matched with interventions as they progress through the stages of change. It is not appropriate to give the whole range of interventions to every client (although some may require this), and clients should be individually matched with those components of the intervention that are most appropriate to his or her needs. Even within modules, not all approaches will be appropriate for every client. Miller (1989) suggests that it is prudent to try the least intensive intervention first, since this is least intrusive and places fewer demands upon resources. Indeed, brief interventions, such as advice

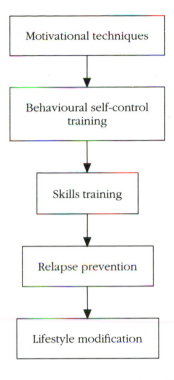

Figure 5.1   *Modules of intervention (McMurran and Hollin, 1993).*

from health professionals, can be sufficient to effect change and, since resources are thus used efficiently and economically, this enables more clients to receive a service (Bien *et al.*, 1993). If the least intensive intervention fails, then there remains the opportunity to step up to the next level of intensity, and the most intensive interventions should be reserved for those who need them.

Before going on to describe these interventions, it is appropriate to mention goals of intervention. Some clients may want to abstain, others may want to cut down, and others may wish to continue drinking or drug use but avoid associated problems. Again, it is important to match the client with appropriate goals. A young person who is drinking heavily and getting into trouble with the law may benefit from aiming to moderate his or her drinking, or even just aiming to change social and situational factors, such as drinking companions and drinking venues. On the other hand, for a drinker who has physical problems, such as liver damage, the most appropriate goal may be abstinence. Negotiating goals with the client is important in order to engage the client in intervention. If the professional forces his or her goals on the client, this is likely to hinder the change process. Of course, the professional may accept the client's goals as a provisional agreement to be renegotiated later.

Where drinking is concerned, the goal of moderation is most likely to be achieved by younger people, particularly females, with a lower severity of dependence upon alcohol, who believe that control is possible, and who are psychologically and socially stable (Rosenberg, 1993). Abstinence is the goal indicated for older, more dependent drinkers, who see themselves as 'alcoholics', and who do not have stable jobs, homes and social networks. Since drug use is against the law, some therapists may see abstinence as the only ethical goal, however, others may take a more pragmatic approach. Controlled drug use can lead to fewer risks and problems, and, most importantly, the issue of HIV transmission must be addressed by changing drug administration practices.

Motivational Techniques

Motivating people to change is a major issue in interventions for addictive behaviours. Change is considered desirable for those who are seen by others to drink or use drugs too much for their own good, or who cause problems to others as a consequence of their drinking or drug use. Of course, the person of concern may not view the situation in quite the same way, and change is not necessarily on his or her agenda. This situation could be interpreted as the drinker or drug user exercising his or her right to choose what to do, but some people see it as 'denial' of a problem. That is, everyone can see that a problem exists, except the person who 'has' the problem.

In the USA, the traditional response to 'denial' has been to confront the 'alcoholic' or 'addict'. Miller and Rollnick (1991), in their book on motivational interviewing, cite an extreme example of confrontation from the *Wall Street Journal*. This took the form of a surprise meeting organized by a group of colleagues to confront a business executive about his drinking. They ganged up and criticized his work, and threatened to fire him unless he went for help. When the executive tried to deny his drinking problem, he was told to 'Shut up and listen. Alcoholics are liars so we don't want to hear what you have to say.' Miller and Rollnick point out that a confrontational approach such as this actually elicits denial; it is quite normal for the victim to respond to an antagonistic approach by defending his or her position. In counselling or therapy

Table 5.2   *Self-motivational statements*

> *Problem recognition*
>   'I suppose my drinking does cause problems at home.'
>   'I spend all my money on heroin, and the family suffers.'
> *Expression of concern*
>   'I'm worried about how much I drink.'
>   'I'm afraid I might become ill.'
> *Intention to change*
>   'I want to get back in control.'
>   'I think I should cut down.'
> *Optimism about change*
>   'I know I can cut down.'
>   'Stopping won't be easy, but I'm sure I can cope.'

for addictions, this often has the effect of exacerbating the problem. Miller (1983) suggests that the key principle is that a person's beliefs and attitudes are shaped by what they say: 'I learn what I believe as I hear myself talk.' If the client is forced into a position of defending his or her behaviour, this serves to strengthen his or her arguments *for* that behaviour. The likely outcome is that the problem behaviour will not change, and it may even get worse. This is clearly contrary to the therapeutic aim.

From this position, Miller and his colleagues developed a strategy known as motivational interviewing. He suggests that denial is not a characteristic of the client. Indeed, what most people bring to therapy is ambivalence, in that both the positive and negative aspects of the behaviour are apparent, as are the costs and benefits of change. The therapist must manage this ambivalence in such a way as to enhance motivation to change. This is done by placing the client in the position of stating the negative aspects of the behaviour and making the case for change. In this way, the principle contained in the statement 'I learn what I believe as I hear myself talk' acts to good effect.

In essence, the therapist attempts to elicit *self-motivational statements* from the client. Self-motivational statements are of four types: problem recognition, expression of concern, intention to change, and optimism about change (Miller and Rollnick, 1991). Examples of these are given in Table 5.2.

A motivational interviewing style is one where the therapist accepts the client as a responsible person, capable of making rational decisions about his or her drinking or drug use, and capable of making efforts to change. This empathic, optimistic and helpful stance contributes to enhancing the client's self-esteem. The therapist raises the client's awareness of personal risk by providing information, commenting

Table 5.3   *Techniques of motivational interviewing*

Avoiding labelling: The therapist avoids labelling the client an 'alcoholic' or 'addict'. If the client does not share the professional's 'diagnosis', then a situation of confrontation and denial will follow, and this will militate against change. In addition, these labels may imply that the client's problems are beyond his or her personal control. The client may infer the need for certain types of 'treatment', such as drugs or long-term intensive therapy, which may not appeal.

Asking evocative questions: The therapist assumes that the client recognizes the problems and that change is desirable. A question based on this assumption is 'What concerns you about your drinking?' This is more likely to elicit a self-motivational statement than a closed question such as 'Are you concerned about your drinking?'

Listing advantages and disadvantages: In order to increase the client's awareness of self and the problem, he or she is asked to list the advantages and disadvantages of the behaviour, both in the short term and the long term.

Acknowledging the positives: The therapist acknowledges the positive effects of the behaviour for the client to elicit a 'Yes, but . . .' response. For example, 'Drinking seems to help you cope with your worries', which might elicit 'Yes, but it's expensive, and adds money worries to the rest of my problems.'

Asking the client to elaborate upon self-motivational statements: When a self-motivational statement is elicited, asking for further information can add other self-motivational statements.

Voicing the client's doubts: When the client defends his or her behaviour, the therapist can issue a paradoxical challenge, placing the client in the position of persuading the therapist of the benefits of change. For example, 'I'm happy with my drug taking; it's my girlfriend who complains' could be challenged by saying 'Perhaps you shouldn't change just for your girlfriend.'

Reversing roles: The therapist and client enact each other's roles; the client-acting-therapist makes the case for change.

Summarizing: At intervals, the therapist summarizes what the client has said, taking care to emphasize self-motivational statements and reframe self-defeating statements. An example of reframing would be to change 'I've tried to stop before, but I can't do it' into 'You're obviously motivated to change since you've tried to stop in the past, so perhaps you just need advice on the best way to go about it.'

on faulty beliefs, and drawing attention to inconsistencies in the client's explanation of his or her behaviour. This highlights the discrepancy between the desired goal and the client's present state. The therapist also suggests a range of alternative goals and interventions that are open to the client. Negotiating with the client what might produce the best outcome contributes to enhancing the client's self-efficacy. Specific techniques used in motivational interviewing are presented in Table 5.3.

Motivational interviewing aims to bring the client to the point of making a decision to change. Throughout the motivational interview (or, more likely, series of interviews), well-timed assessment, feedback and advice are all helpful. In *assessment*, the problem behaviour is examined in detail, using a variety of methods, as shown in Table 5.4.

For some clients, motivational interviewing that includes feedback

Table 5.4   *Methods of assessment*

Direct observation: In some cases, it may be possible to observe the client in context to gather the necessary information. Often, however, there are ethical problems in doing so; some of the behaviours of interest are against the law, and observation involves considerable intrusion into the client's life. Direct observation is usually impractical in that the therapist cannot afford the time to watch a client in action. In addition, it is unlikely that the client would behave in his or her normal manner while being observed by a 'fly on the wall'.

Interviews: In almost all cases the therapist will gather information in interview, asking about the development of the problem, present status of the problem, and related issues such as relationships, work and leisure pursuits.

Diaries: Clients may be asked to keep a diary of their drinking and drug use to measure what is used, how much, when, and under what circumstances.

Analogue assessments: The client may be asked to role play a situation in an approximation to real-life conditions, using props and other actors. The therapist can then assess the client's performance, for example his or her ability to say 'no' to drink or drugs when under pressure from peers. Actual alcohol is sometimes used in analogue assessments to measure resistance to temptation and speed of drinking.

Psychometric tests: A number of questionnaires have been developed to measure levels of dependence on alcohol and drugs, motivation to change, and confidence about being able to resist consumption in certain situations.

Neuropsychological tests: Tests designed to examine cognitive functioning and organic brain damage can be useful in determining goals and methods of intervention.

Biological tests: Blood, breath and urine tests may be taken to assess the amount of alcohol or drugs in the body. Blood tests and biopsies can measure organic damage as a consequence of alcohol and drug use.

---

and advice may be a sufficient intervention. Miller and Sovereign (1989) describe a Drinker's Check-Up, comprising two visits to a clinic for assessment and feedback using motivational interviewing techniques. In comparison with clients on a waiting list control, their alcohol consumption was significantly reduced at a six-week follow-up. The Drinker's Check-Up has been found more effective when conducted in a motivational style, as opposed to a directive, confrontational fashion. While some clients may benefit from motivational interviewing that includes assessment, personal feedback and advice, others will require help with the action stage of change.

Behavioural Self-Control Training

Behavioural self-control training, abbreviated to BSCT, is the process of teaching people the skills and strategies they need to control their own behaviour. Most people do not employ a scientific approach when making attempts to change, and it helps to teach them to specify the behaviour that requires change, identify its antecedents and consequences, and formulate an action plan. Mahoney and Thoresen (1974) describe this as teaching the individual to become a 'personal scientist' by systematic self-observation, analysing personal data, testing out techniques for change, and evaluating outcome.

BSCT brings behaviour under control by focusing attention on it, reducing automatic processing, and reintroducing controlled processing. *Automatic processing* is where little conscious attention is paid to a behaviour and its execution is not dependent upon a continual decision making process (Kanfer and Gaelick, 1986). Where many everyday behaviours are concerned, automatic processing is highly efficient. Practised drivers, for example, do not need to deliberate about every manoeuvre they make during a journey and the business of driving is facilitated by automatic processing. *Controlled processing*, by contrast, requires constant attention to the surroundings and the behaviour to gather and process information which is then used in making decisions about what to do next. This operates when learning new behaviours; for example, upon starting to drive a car nothing comes automatically, except perhaps the ability to stall the engine. Where problem behaviours are concerned, an automatic chain of responses triggered by environmental or internal cues is not beneficial, and there is a need to 'deautomize' troublesome behaviours, thus bringing them under control.

BSCT begins with *self-monitoring*, where the client systematically studies the behaviour, its antecedents, and its consequences. This is typically done by keeping a diary of the type shown in Figure 5.2. Clients are then taught to study their diaries to look for factors that may be associated with drinking or drug use, such as the day of the week, the time of day and particular places, people, activities or moods. Self-monitoring is the foundation of *discrimination training*. That is, the individual must learn to discriminate the antecedent stimuli that lead to certain behavioural responses, and the consequences that maintain those responses. Only with this knowledge can the client then utilize the other skills of self-control (Brigham, 1982). Indeed, in some cases these skills follow without further intervention; the *reactivity effect* is the name given to the observation that self-monitoring alone can lead to behaviour change.

Self-monitoring leads on to *goal setting*, where the client sets limits on his or her drinking or drug use. These goals are stated specifically, in terms of setting maximum consumption limits, restrictions on days or

Day	Time	Place	Who with	Why start	Type of drug	Amount used	Cost	Consequences
Monday								
Tuesday								
Wednesday								
Thursday								
Friday								
Saturday								
Sunday								

Figure 5.2   *Self-monitoring diary*

times when consumption is personally permitted, and the amount of money allowed for spending on drink or drugs. Precision is important, since many people simply express a vague intention to cut down, but have no concrete idea of what this means. Continued self-monitoring enables clients to check their actual consumption against the goals they have set.

The next step is to change the antecedents to the behaviour by *setting rules*. Drinking and drug use may be viewed as the culmination of a chain of events, each of which triggers the next. An example of a chain might be contacting friends on Saturday afternoon, arranging to meet for a drink, going to the pub, having a few drinks and then moving on to a club. Rules may be targeted at breaking the chain at an early stage, for example by arranging to spend Saturday night in an activity which does not involve drinking. This is called *decisional self-control*, in that a single choice is made to remove a tempting goal and, once this choice has been made, it is difficult to reverse (Kanfer and Gaelick, 1986). Rules may also alter immediate antecedents, which is known as *stimulus control*. Taking smoking as an example here, the would-be non-smoker could reduce the temptation to have a cigarette by removing from the house all visual cues related to smoking, that is disposing of cigarettes, ashtrays and lighters. Situational factors implicated in the desire to smoke could be changed, such as engaging in an absorbing activity immediately after eating a meal instead of having a cup of coffee, which used to be accompanied by a cigarette. Both decisional self-control strategies and stimulus control strategies can be listed as a set of personal rules to be followed in the effort to achieve the goals of limited drinking or drug use. Examples of personal rules would be 'I will drink only on Thursday and Saturday. I will not drink before 8 p.m. I will not keep alcohol in the house.'

The behaviour itself is also addressed in BSCT, particularly where moderation is the goal. This involves *rate control* strategies. Kanfer and Gaelick (1986) call this *protracted self-control* in that resistance to temptation must be exercised over a period of time. Rate control strategies for moderating alcohol consumption when in a drinking situation might include choosing low alcohol drinks, taking a half pint instead of a pint of beer, and learning to sip drinks slowly.

Contingency management involves altering the consequences of behaviour, setting up a system of *self-reward* for adhering to one's goals, and, to a lesser degree, *self-punishment* for failure to adhere to one's goals. Rewards may be material goods, for example buying a special treat with the money saved from reduced drinking or drug taking, or they may be positive self-statements, which are simply giving oneself a pat on the back for doing well, for example 'I kept to my limit, and this is good progress.' Pleasant activities may also be rearranged to make these contingent upon successful goal attainment, for example allowing oneself to watch a favourite television programme only if the day's goal has been achieved. Self-punishment for failure to stick to one's goal might, for example, be to do a necessary but unpleasant task such as tidying the attic, cleaning the cooker or digging the garden.

BSCT has been shown to be effective with problem drinkers (Miller, 1978). It works well both when the client works with a therapist (Miller *et al.*, 1981; Miller and Taylor, 1980) and when the client works alone, using a self-help manual (Miller and Baca, 1983; Heather *et al.*, 1986). The contingency management component of BSCT has been successfully used in interventions with drug users, although these are usually administered by the therapist, rather than by the client himself or herself (Tucker *et al.*, 1992). The incentives used include allowing clients personal control over their dosage and administration of methadone, and asking the client to deposit a sum of money with the therapist who returns some of this each week if the client has been drug-free (Kleber, 1989).

The techniques of BSCT may be seen as temporary devices, used by the client only until new behaviours become well established. Maintenance of these new behaviours may well depend upon acquiring new skills, which is addressed in the next component of intervention.

Skills Training

When attempts are made to change drinking and drug use, a number of obstacles may be met. First, interactions with other people may present problems, for example coping with peer pressure to drink or use drugs, or learning to socialize confidently without the aid of alcohol or drugs. These issues are dealt with in *social skills training*. Second, changing one's habits may give rise to new problems, such as how to fill the time now that less of it is devoted to drinking or drug use, or how to cope with unpleasant emotions without resorting to 'self-medication'. These issues are addressed in *problem solving training*. Third, *stress management training* can help in cases where substances have been used to manage tension or anxiety. These three interventions will be described in turn.

Social Skills Training

Social skills are essentially those necessary for communication with other people. These skills are both verbal and non-verbal. Verbal skills include not only what is said, but also the manner in which it is said, in terms of volume, tone, pitch and speed of speech. Non-verbal skills contain elements such as body posture, gestures and facial expression. For good communication, verbal and non-verbal skills should show consistency. Refusing a request, for example, does not sound sincere if the person saying 'No' makes the vowel-sound too long, looks downwards and fidgets. In addition to consistency, good social skills require sensitivity to the social situation, listening to what other people have to say, reading their non-verbal signals and making an appropriate response.

The situations that people find difficult vary from person to person, and the assessment of specific problem areas occurs prior to social skills training. The kinds of skills typically taught in interventions aimed

Table 5.5   *Social skills programme (after Monti, et al., 1989)*

Starting conversations
Giving and receiving compliments
Non-verbal communication
Talking about feelings
Listening skills
Assertiveness
Giving criticism
Receiving criticism
Receiving criticism about drinking
Drink refusal skills
Refusing requests
Communication in close relationships
Building social support networks

at reducing drinking are illustrated in the programme designed by Monti *et al.* (1989) presented in Table 5.5.

The method used to teach social skills is *role-play*. The aim is to act out an anticipated situation in order to practise skills and get feedback about performance. This is very similar to actors rehearsing a play; they may try out several ways of saying their lines to see which works best, and they will receive advice from the director. The problematic social situation is first discussed by the client and the therapist so that both are familiar with the likely scenario. The main components thereafter are: *modelling*, where a demonstration of a competent performance is given; *rehearsal*, where the client practises the part; and *feedback*, where the client and therapist discuss the performance and identify ways of improvement.

A number of studies have shown that social skills training is effective in helping problem drinkers reduce their alcohol consumption. In his review of this literature, Chaney (1989) concludes that 'skills training has received sufficient empirical evaluation to be ensured a permanent role in alcoholism treatment' (p. 219). Outcome studies of skills training programmes for drug users are lacking, but it is reasonable to assume that social skills training would also be effective with this group (Tucker *et al.*, 1992).

Problem Solving Training

Problem solving derives from the work of D'Zurilla and Goldfried (1971), who view problem behaviours, including addiction, as ineffective means of coping with problematic situations. They define problem solving as a process which '(a) makes available a variety of potentially effective response alternatives for dealing with the problematic situation, and (b) increases the probability of selecting the most effective response from among these various alternatives' (p. 108).

Problem solving training has five separate stages. *Orientation* involves teaching people to recognize a problem when one occurs, and then to stop and think about a solution. Attention is focused on 'bad feelings', that is any unpleasant state, which could be anger, anxiety, depression, boredom, withdrawal symptoms, or urges to drink or use drugs. Instead of ignoring these bad feelings, or simply enduring them, they become cues to move to the next stage, that is *problem definition and goal setting*. The problem should be defined clearly by describing the facts of the situation and identifying the factors that are making the situation problematic, then realistic goals should be set. The next stage is the *generation of alternatives*, that is looking creatively for a variety of strategies which will attain these goals. *Decision making and action* is the stage where the best options are selected and an action plan is formed. Finally, there is *evaluation* of the success of the action plan. Where goals have been met, then the problem solving process is complete; if goals have not been achieved, then the process may begin again, perhaps focusing on issues which have prevented success by taking these to be the next problem. In practice, problem solving can be taught by posing six questions:

1 Bad feelings?
2 What is my problem?
3 What are my goals?
4 What are my options?
5 What is my plan?
6 How did I do?

A worked example is presented in Table 5.6.

Chaney *et al.* (1978) compared problem solving training with a placebo control (discussion groups) and a no-intervention control with men in an in-patient alcohol treatment programme. At the one-year follow-up, the problem solving group was compared with the two control groups combined and found to be significantly more improved on measures of number of days drunk, total number of drinks and mean length of drinking periods.

Table 5.6 *Problem solving*

1 *Bad feelings?*
Tiredness, stress

2 *What is my problem?*
I have exams to work for and I'm behind schedule. I've spent too long trying to understand a concept in chemistry which I don't understand. I'm worried I might fail. I've been getting away from the pressure by going to the bar most nights. I've been drinking too much and staying up too late.

3 *What are my goals?*
a To get up-to-date with my revision.
b To pass my exams.

4 *What are my options?*	*Pros*	*Cons*
a Drop out of college.	Less pressure.	Fewer career options.
b Ask the chemistry lecturer for help.	Sort out confusion.	She might think I didn't go to her lecture.
c Go to the bar only on Saturday night.	Have one good night out. Get to bed early rest of the week.	Will miss talking to friends during the week.
d Go to the bar some nights, but drink soft drinks.	Will see my friends. Will not get drunk. Will be able to work next day.	Will be tempted to drink. Might still stay up too late.
e Buy wine to drink in my room.	Would help me relax. Would go to bed early.	Would get drunk.
f Relax some other way, e.g. go swimming, watch TV.	Would not need to drink so much.	Would take up work time.
g Go home to my parents' house to study.	I'd be looked after. No distractions. No drinking.	I'd get bored. No access to library.

5 *What is my plan?*
a Ask the chemistry lecturer for help.
b Have one night out drinking on Saturday.
c Go out on Wednesday night but do not drink.
d Watch TV for one hour before going to bed.

6 *How did I do?*
The chemistry lecturer helped me understand the problem. I got on with the rest of my revision after that. For the past two weeks I have been drinking only on Saturday nights. I have not been watching TV to relax. I still go to the bar most nights, but I do not drink alcohol. This way, I still meet my friends, but I don't feel tired and hungover the next day. I am almost back on schedule with my revision. I feel more relaxed and confident about my exams.

Stress Management Training

Stockwell and Town (1989) suggest that there are three components to interventions designed to help people gain control of their reactions to stress:

1 altering the environment to reduce the frequency and severity of external stressors;
2 altering the person's perception of a stressor; and
3 using active coping strategies.

The first step is to identify what exactly is creating the tension, then, having identified the cause, steps may sometimes be taken to eliminate or attenuate the stressor. For example, domestic issues such as who takes out the rubbish, how long the bathroom may be occupied, and what volume of noise is acceptable may be tackled through negotiating house rules. Social skills and problem solving skills can be useful here.

Stress may be created by the way a person thinks about an event rather than the fact of the event itself. Distorting the facts through negative or irrational thinking can lead to tension, anxiety and other unpleasant emotions. Negative thinking should be substituted by more positive and reasonable thoughts. Monti *et al.* (1989) describe a three-step procedure for changing negative thinking:

1 catch yourself thinking negatively;
2 stop yourself; and
3 challenge the negative thoughts and substitute positive thinking.

An example might be where the initiating event was passing one's boss in a corridor at work and the boss did not smile when she said good morning. Negative or irrational thinking might turn this into rejection, implied criticism and fear – 'My boss does not like me'; 'My boss did not like my last report'; 'I will lose my job'. Negative thoughts such as these should be identified and challenged, then replaced with more positive thinking. 'It is possible that the boss was preoccupied with her own thoughts'; 'I will ask for an appointment to discuss the report and find out what she really thinks'; 'Just because she did not smile at me does not mean that I am going to get the sack.'

Using the above techniques is unlikely to eliminate stress altogether and coping strategies should be part of a person's behavioural

Table 5.7 *Muscle relaxation exercises*

First make sure you are lying or sitting comfortably. Muscle relaxation involves tensing and stretching of the muscles, followed by relaxation. These exercises should be carried out slowly and gently. Concentrate on the difference between tension and relaxation.

First stretch your legs and point your toes. Hold this position for a few seconds, then relax. Now press your knees together, hold and relax. Pull in your stomach, hold and relax. Arch your lower back, hold and relax. Press your elbows into your sides, hold and relax. Stretch your arms, spread your fingers, hold and relax. Shrug your shoulders, hold and relax. Stretch your neck by bending your head to the right, then the left and relax. Raise your eyebrows, hold and relax. Scowl, hold and relax.

Now attend to each part of your body in turn, making sure there is no tension in your muscles. Relax your feet, your calves, your thighs, your stomach, your back, your chest, your hands, your arms, your shoulders and your face.

Sit quietly with your eyes closed for a few moments and concentrate on your breathing. Each time you breathe out, say the word 'relax' quietly to yourself. When you feel ready, open your eyes, stretch your body, and continue your usual activities calmly.

---

repertoire. The ability to relax is one useful coping skill. There are a number of possible components to relaxation. First, there are *relaxing activities*, such as going for a walk, soaking in the bath or listening to music. Clients may be advised to programme such activities into their daily routine. Second, *muscle relaxation* is a method of coping with stress based on the premise that muscle tension is closely related to anxiety, and that the experience of anxiety will be reduced if tense muscles can be made to relax. Clients may be taught techniques for muscle relaxation, as shown in Table 5.7. Once physically relaxed, *imagery* may be introduced. Here, the client is asked to imagine a calming object or scene. Typical images used in relaxation are to focus thoughts on a flickering candle flame, bubbles rising in a glass of carbonated water, or white clouds drifting across a blue sky. A particular favourite is to ask the client to imagine himself or herself lying in the soft sand on a deserted beach feeling the sun warming the skin and listening to the gentle sound of waves lapping on the shore.

Rohsenow *et al.* (1986) found that a stress management intervention with college students reduced alcohol consumption at the six-month follow-up, with the most anxious and heaviest drinkers showing the greatest change. Reviews of the area have concluded that stress management procedures can help in reducing drinking and drug use, but only for those clients who are experiencing anxiety (Miller and Hester, 1986; Tucker *et al.*, 1992). This makes obvious sense, and clients should be selected for skills training in any of the areas described

Table 5.8 *Determinants of relapse (after Marlatt, 1985b)*

1 *Intrapersonal determinants*
   a Unpleasant emotions: Experiencing frustration, anger, loneliness, boredom, worry and other negative emotional states.
   b Physical discomfort: Experiencing physical withdrawal or other discomfort such as pain, illness and fatigue.
   c Pleasant emotions: Feeling happy, excited, pleased and other positive emotional states.
   d Testing personal control: Wishing to test one's ability to engage in controlled or moderate use.
   e Urges and temptations: Feeling 'cravings', or unexpectedly finding oneself in a situation which presents the opportunity to indulge.
2 *Interpersonal determinants*
   a Conflict: Having arguments, fights or disagreements with other people.
   b Social pressure: Being urged to indulge or seeing other people indulge and feeling the need to join in.
   c Pleasant times: Use of a substance to enhance pleasant times, such as a romantic or sexual situation, a night on the town or a celebration.

above only where they are deficient in the particular coping skills targeted in the programme.

Relapse Prevention

Mark Twain once claimed that stopping smoking is easy – he had done it hundreds of times. This illustrates one major problem in attempting to change addictive behaviours, that is high rates of relapse. Clients often manage to control their addictions in the short term, but have difficulty entering into the maintenance stage of change. The problem of relapse has been given considerable attention, leading to the development of the intervention programme known as relapse prevention. This is designed to help clients anticipate and cope with situations that might precipitate a relapse.

The first step is to identify those situations that present a risk for relapse. Marlatt (1985b) lists eight common determinants of relapse within two categories: intrapersonal and interpersonal (Table 5.8). Of these, unpleasant emotions, interpersonal conflict and social pressure account for most relapses, but each person will have a different risk profile. This must be assessed along with the individual's coping skills for dealing with high risk situations.

Coping with Temptation

In avoiding relapse, the client must be taught to cope with temptation. The first step is to put the experience of desire into perspective. The desire to drink or use drugs is to be expected from time to time; it is a normal experience for those attempting change. Feelings of desire should become the cue for activating coping strategies, which may be applied until the desire dissipates.

There are three main strategies for coping with desire. The client may use *positive self-statements* to strengthen resolve. This involves saying to oneself statements such as:

I expected to feel like having a drink, and it's not that bad really.

I expected to want drugs again, but I don't need to give in to the feeling.

I feel tempted, but I won't let the feeling beat me.

The next step is a *decision review*. Commitment to change is likely to be enhanced where the client keeps in mind the reasons that prompted the decision to change in the first place. A decision review involves looking at the pros and cons of indulging in the behaviour versus not indulging in the behaviour, both in the short term and the long term. Focusing on both the immediate and the delayed consequences encourages the client to address what Marlatt (1985a) calls the PIG – the problem of immediate gratification. This is the tendency, where addictive behaviours are concerned, to be attracted by the immediate rewards at the expense of the longer term costs.

Although it is useful to recognize the desire to indulge, make positive self-statements and review one's decision to change, *distraction* from the feelings of desire soon becomes necessary. The best distracting activities are those that are incompatible with the behaviour one is trying to control. Swimming, for example, is incompatible with most other activities – smoking, drinking, drug use and so on. An activity that requires concentration may also help, for example reading, doing crossword puzzles or baking a cake. Marlatt (1985a) cautions against 'seemingly irrelevant decisions' or SIDs. These are activities which on the surface appear to be distracting, but actually place the person in a

Table 5.9   *Covert modelling script*

It is Saturday night. You have been out drinking with Dave, Alice and Nick. You are all in Nick's flat having another beer. Dave begins to roll a joint. When you see him doing this, you feel desperate for a smoke, but you have decided to stop. You say to yourself, 'I knew I'd feel the urge to smoke, but I don't have to give in.' That makes you feel more able to resist.

Dave smokes first, then passes the joint to Alice. Alice passes it on to you. You shake your head and say, 'No, thanks.' Alice says it's really good stuff, but you say no again. Dave gives you a funny look.

You start up a conversation about music, and the awkward moment passes. You feel pleased that you have stuck to your decision.

situation of greater temptation. Examples of SIDs are: the decision to go shopping in the supermarket where the drinks section must be encountered on the route to the checkout; going to the newsagent to buy a magazine knowing that the newsagent also sells cigarettes; or going to visit a friend when that friend is known to smoke cannabis.

Covert Modelling

Covert modelling is a technique for 'practising' coping skills in one's imagination. The client is asked to imagine encountering a high-risk situation with which he or she copes successfully. The situation to be imagined is worked out in detail by the client and the therapist. A script is then prepared and read aloud to the client, who imagines himself or herself in that situation, saying, doing and feeling everything as vividly as possible. A sample script is presented in Table 5.9. A covert modelling script is personal, describes real-life situations and contains specific details about the context, the people present and the behaviour. The coping strategy is emphasized, as are the good feelings that follow success.

Coping with Lapses

In relapse prevention, it is important to acknowledge that setbacks may occur. In coping with setbacks, the essence is to avoid the 'goal violation effect' (GVE) or the 'abstinence violation effect' (AVE). These are similar phenomena that apply to moderation and abstinence goals respectively. These violation effects describe the observation that when a lapse occurs, this often leads to a full-blown relapse. A dieter, for example, who eats one chocolate biscuit may not stop at one but go on to eat the whole packet. The belief, common amongst those who adhere to the disease model of alcoholism, that one drink triggers an uncontrollable urge to drink more may actually contribute to the AVE; that is, for the drinker who holds this notion, it is likely to become a self-fulfilling prophecy.

Marlatt (1985c) proposes that violation of personal goals should be *reframed*. This entails defining failures as a lapse or a slip, rather than a relapse. Lapses are viewed as learning experiences, thus empowering the client to look for new coping skills. The client is encouraged to look for the cause of a lapse in external circumstances (external attribution), such as encountering a high-risk situation, instead of attributing the lapse to stable personal factors (internal attribution), such as 'having no willpower'. Internal attributions of causality can lead the person to see himself or herself as a lost cause and give up trying to change. By contrast, external attributions of causality prompt the client to identify what the problem was and what could be done to guard against a future lapse, should the same situation occur again.

Marlatt also suggests providing the client with *emergency procedures* that may be applied immediately, should a lapse occur. They will serve to limit the extent of the lapse. The following instructions, which would be presented to a drinking client, are an example of a set of emergency procedures: Stop drinking; put your glass down; remind yourself of why you wanted to cut down your drinking; leave the high-risk situation; do something else that you like.

Relapse rehearsal is similar to covert modelling, only it applies to those skills which will help limit the lapse. Here the client is asked to imagine a situation in which a lapse has occurred, followed by successful application of the emergency procedures.

Graded Practice

Much of the relapse prevention intervention is aimed at preparing the client to meet risk; up to this point, the client may have been advised to avoid high-risk situations. However, there comes a time when real-life practice is necessary. A hierarchy of risk situations is drawn up for each client, and there is a graded plan of exposure first to the least risky, and then on to progressively more difficult situations. The therapist prepares the client by helping him or her identify likely difficulties and rehearsing the necessary coping skills. The aim here is to develop self-efficacy by allowing the client to experience mastery over a situation.

Marlatt (1985a) recommends that relapse prevention interventions should then move on to addressing broader issues, such as work, use of leisure time and relationships. This enables the client to establish a lifestyle that maintains the behaviour change, rather than continuing to cope with one high-risk situation after another. Lifestyle modification, which is often included within a relapse prevention programme, is addressed next.

In a review of relapse prevention procedures, Mattick and Heather (1993) suggest that this approach is effective when used in combination with other interventions, for example behavioural–marital therapy, and counselling plus drug treatment. It seems to be the case that relapse prevention successfully teaches people to attribute relapse to personally controllable factors, and to take greater personal responsibility for avoiding future relapse, and that this enhances the likelihood of abstinence from alcohol and drugs.

Lifestyle Modification

From studies of those who change their addictive behaviour without help, managing change successfully in the long term depends upon the creation of a new lifestyle (Stall and Biernacki, 1986). Reducing drinking or drug use often requires that the former problematic user avoids certain friends and social venues and find new activities to fill the time previously taken up by drinking or drug use. Unsatisfactory relationships that lead to drinking or drug use or relationships that have been damaged by drinking or drug use may have to be sorted out. Lifestyle modification is a term used for a number of interventions addressing such issues.

One example of a broad-based approach to lifestyle modification is the *community reinforcement approach*. This approach, used with problem drinkers, includes Antabuse prescription, marriage counselling, employment counselling, social skills training and recreational advice. The overall aim is to enable the former drinker to have a meaningful life without alcohol by rearranging the individual's social environment so that it is supportive of sobriety (Sisson and Azrin, 1989). Clients in this programme have been shown to drink on fewer days and spend more days working compared with clients in a hospital treatment programme.

Marital and family therapy is often seen as an important area of intervention for maintaining change. Relationship difficulties can be a contributing factor in substance use, but substance use may also contribute to the deterioration of relationships. In recognition of this, marital therapy (which can also apply to partners who are not married, including lesbians and gay men) and family therapy are often included in intervention. The areas that may be addressed are domestic responsibilities, money management, sex, social activities and communication (Sisson and Azrin, 1989).

Miller and Hester (1986), in their brief review of the effectiveness of marital and family therapy with problem drinkers, conclude that improvements are apparent in the short term, but that these do not endure over time. In addition, the improvements which do accrue relate more to marital adjustment than to drinking. O'Farrell *et al.* (1992) suggest that marital therapy may be useful in promoting 'relationship stability during the long and arduous period of recovery from alcoholism' (p. 530).

Other Psychological Interventions

The modular programme outlined above contains interventions based mainly on operant conditioning and social learning theories. There are other important interventions based on classical conditioning theory that deserve attention – cue exposure and response prevention, aversion therapy and covert sensitization. Despite evidence for the effectiveness of these interventions, they remain relatively unpopular in practice. Interventions based on expectancy theory are at the stage of being developed in practice, but are likely to become important components of intervention in future, and a brief description of expectancy challenge is presented here. Psychotherapy and counselling approaches are also mentioned.

Cue Exposure and Response Prevention

Resistance to temptation can be strengthened by cue exposure and response prevention. Here, the therapist exposes the client to the cues that trigger the desire to indulge, but prevents the behaviour actually occurring. This may extinguish the desire by breaking down the association between the cues and the response. Alternatively, this intervention may take effect by changing the client's efficacy expectations; that is, the person's beliefs about his or her ability to cope in high-risk situations are enhanced. The actual cues to which the client may be exposed range from simple objects, for example a bottle of alcohol or injecting equipment, to complex social situations, for example a pub or a party. Rohsenow *et al.* (1991), in their review of cue reactivity, note that cue exposure with response prevention reduced alcohol consumption in problem drinkers, and reduced cravings and withdrawal in opiate and cocaine users.

Aversion Therapy

Aversion therapy is where stimuli related to substance use, for example the sight or taste of alcohol, are paired with an unpleasant experience, such as chemically induced nausea or an electric shock. Aversion therapy depends upon the repeated pairing of substance-related stimuli with unpleasant experiences to produce a conditioned aversion to the substance of addiction, thereby decreasing substance use.

Where chemical aversion (induced nausea) is concerned, there is difficulty in controlling the onset and severity of the response, therefore electric shock is sometimes used. However, nausea-inducing drugs may be more effective because nausea is more naturally linked with the ingestion of substances compared to the experience of an electric shock. A typical procedure for aversion therapy is described by Elkins (1991). The subject, who has been asked to avoid eating solids for six hours before the intervention, is given a salt water drink. This drink provides the material to be vomited, but also contains the emetic substance. Nausea is experienced within a few minutes. The subject is repeatedly given alcoholic drinks over a 20–30 minute period, and each drink is returned as vomit.

In their review of aversion therapies for alcohol problems, Miller and Hester (1986) conclude that these are effective in suppressing drinking behaviour. The problems associated with aversion therapy are first ethical issues surrounding this unpleasant form of intervention, and second the fact that clients frequently drop out of such programmes. Because of these problems, the type of aversion therapy known as covert sensitization is much more commonly used.

Covert Sensitization

Covert sensitization is a type of aversion therapy where imaginary aversive scenes are linked with the addictive behaviour. The client is asked to relax then follow a script read aloud by the therapist that entails imagining as vividly as possible some unpleasant event occurring immediately after the behaviour targeted for change. Where drinking is concerned, the script might involve imagining drinking, with consequent feelings of nausea and vomiting, including graphic descriptions of the physical sensations of retching and heaving, and the smell and appearance of the vomit. Elkins (1980) worked with a sample of in-patient alcoholics, and found that conditioned nausea could not be induced in all of his subjects. Where conditioned nausea was developed, those subjects showed significantly extended periods of post-treatment abstinence in comparison with subjects who did not develop conditioned nausea.

The induction of nausea is an effective unconditioned stimulus to pair with drinking, the conditioned stimulus, since taste aversions are readily formed when nausea is experienced. Other addictive behaviours may require aversion via different modalities. As a prison psychologist, I once worked with a machine gambler whose habit was getting him into serious trouble with the law in that he was stealing in order to gamble. This young man had a revulsion for snakes, and covert sensitization included asking him to imagine hitting the jackpot, but instead of coins pouring from the slot, the machine produced lots of wriggling snakes. At the one year follow-up, this client was no longer playing gaming machines.

Expectancy Challenge

Challenging alcohol outcome expectancies has been included as a component of some intervention programmes. Here, the client is given a drink that he or she believes to contain alcohol, although it does not. A task is then carried out and performance is discussed afterwards. The effects of the drink on task performance cannot be put down to alcohol since none was consumed, therefore the role of outcome expectancies is highlighted. This procedure can be used to challenge common but disadvantageous expectancies, for example that having one drink makes you feel like drinking more.

Baer *et al.* (1991) used expectancy challenge in an alcohol skills-training programme for college students. In a simulated bar setting, subjects were given a non-alcoholic drink that they were told contained alcohol. Afterwards, subjects were asked to describe the effects alcohol had on them, and to say how confident they were that they had consumed alcohol. After revealing the truth, the therapist's discussion focused on the psychological effects versus the pharmacological effects of alcohol. Overall, the intervention was effective in reducing alcohol consumption, but the effectiveness of the expectancy challenge component was not examined separately.

An experiment by Darkes and Goldman (1993), although not a clinical intervention, is instructive in examining the effects of expectancy challenge. Their subjects were male college students who were moderate to heavy drinkers. These subjects were allocated to one of three conditions: expectancy challenge, a traditional alcohol education programme or assessment only. The expectancy challenge intervention consisted of asking subjects to consume a drink. Some drinks contained alcohol and others did not, but the subjects did not know who was drinking what. The group was then asked to engage in a task (a word game in one session and a debate in the second session), after which they were asked to identify who had consumed alcohol and who had consumed the placebo drink. All subjects made some errors in identification, and after revealing this, the experimenters held a discussion about the role of outcome expectancies in drinking and related behaviour. Although no pressure was put upon any subject to reduce alcohol consumption, those in the expectancy challenge group showed a decrease, whereas those in the other two groups actually increased their consumption over the month of the experiment. Positive outcome expectancies were shown to reduce in the expectancy challenge group, but not in the other two groups, which supports the notion that alcohol consumption is mediated by expectancies. As the authors say, this experiment is not sufficient to allow unbounded enthusiasm for expectancy challenge as a therapeutic intervention for problem drinkers, but it does indicate that further work needs to be done to develop this area.

Psychotherapy

Psychotherapy takes a number of different forms, for example the psychoanalytic approaches based on the works of Freud, Jung and others. These therapies are non-directive in that the client is helped to explore his or her problems to gain insight and self-knowledge, and change may ensue from this self-awareness. Psychotherapy may be conducted with individual clients or in groups.

Craig (1993) comments that

> psychotherapy has not been considered the treatment of choice with substance abusers for several reasons: (a) Many believed that drug addicts do not have the introspective and reflective capacity that is required for psychotherapy to be effective; (b) drug addicts appear to have problems in forming an authentic therapeutic alliance because of sociopathic traits; and (c) environmental variables and internal drug-conditioned cues seem to have a more powerful effect on drug addict behaviour than can be overcome with psychotherapy. (p. 186)

Miller and Hester (1986), in their review of psychotherapy for alcohol problems, conclude that there is no persuasive evidence for the effectiveness of these approaches. Evidence from the field of drug intervention is equivocal. Craig (1993) points out that some heroin addicts may be able to benefit from psychotherapy, and it remains to identify for which clients this is appropriate. Research has, in fact, shown that cognitive style has a bearing on how well clients fare in psychotherapy. McLachlan (1972) showed that complex, abstract thinkers showed better outcomes in non-directive therapy for alcohol problems than simplistic, concrete thinkers. The latter fared better with a directive therapist.

Non-Psychological Interventions

Detoxification

Detoxification is the process of taking an individual off a drug. This can be done abruptly ('cold turkey') or gradually under medical or nursing supervision. Drugs may be used to counteract withdrawal symptoms, and attention is paid to the client's general health and well-being. Vitamin and mineral supplements are usually given, since drinkers and drug users are often malnourished. While detoxification will benefit a client, psychological intervention is likely to be needed to help that person develop the skills to maintain change.

Drug Treatments

Three types of drug treatment exist for addiction problems. The first is the use of drugs that alter the effects of the drug of addiction. The antidipsotropic drug disulfiram, usually known by its trade name of Antabuse, has no effect until alcohol is consumed, whereupon an unpleasant physical reaction is experienced – flushing, palpitations and vomiting. The use of antidipsotropic drugs is not the same as aversion therapy. Antabuse has a deterrent effect upon the would-be drinker, perhaps forcing that person into the position where he or she has to learn alternative strategies for coping with a variety of situations, and as such is a form of cue exposure and response prevention (Brewer, 1990). Naltrexone is an opiate antagonist which blocks the effects of opiates, thus robbing them of their pleasurable effects (Ghodse, 1989). This makes heroin use rather pointless. Kleber (1989) notes that supervised administration of the medication is important in that clients left to self-medicate will often not comply with the programme; however it has proved useful with clients who are well motivated to change.

A second category of drug treatment is maintenance prescription. This is the legal supply of an opiate drug, usually methadone, to prevent craving and withdrawal, thus enabling the client to live a normal life and avoid the hazards associated with the black market. Most programmes aim to wean the client gradually off methadone, but many continue on methadone maintenance for years.

Finally, medication may be aimed at treating underlying psychopathology. Many alcohol and drug-dependent clients experience problems, such as anxiety and depression, which can be alleviated by prescribed drugs.

While drug treatments can benefit the client, there is an attendant problem of the possibility of side-effects that may be damaging to the client's health. These treatments may be best viewed as short term measures which need to be augmented by psychological interventions for maintenance of change.

Rehabilitation

Rehabilitation is the 'process of integrating the drinker or drug user into society so that he/she can cope without drugs and can be restored to the best possible level of functioning' (Ghodse, 1989). Rehabilitation is usually conducted in residential placements, such as hostels, where personal counselling is available and where attention is paid to the client's future accommodation, finances, work and support network.

Twelve-step Programmes

The generic name 'twelve-step programmes' applies to a number of self-help groups which have grown from the original Alcoholics Anonymous (AA). The 'twelve steps' are the core of these programmes; those pertaining to AA are presented in Table 5.10. In addition to AA, Room and Greenfield (1993) report the existence in the US of Cocaine Anonymous, Gamblers Anonymous, Marijuana Anonymous, Narcotics Anonymous, Nicotine Anonymous, Overeaters Anonymous, Sexaholics Anonymous, Smokers Anonymous and Workaholics Anonymous, amongst others. Groups also exist to help partners and children of those with addiction problems, for example Al-Anon (mainly for partners of 'alcoholics'), Al-Ateen (for their teenage children) and Adult Children of Alcoholics (Room and Greenfield, 1993).

Twelve-step groups are fellowships of men and women who meet regularly to support each other in their efforts to achieve and maintain abstinence. Groups are run by the members themselves, who are not professional counsellors. They have a spiritual foundation, but are not affiliated with any organized religion. Twelve-step groups operate on the premise that it is essential for the person to admit to being an alcoholic or an addict, and then to relinquish the belief that moderate use is a possibility for them. The difficulties encountered in remaining abstinent, and the discouraging prospect of making a resolution to avoid alcohol or drugs forever, are acknowledged in the slogan 'one

Table 5.10   *The Twelve Steps of Alcoholics Anonymous*

1   We admitted we were powerless over alcohol – that our lives had become un-manageable.
2   Came to believe that a power greater than ourselves could restore us to sanity.
3   Made a decision to turn our will and our lives over to the care of God *as we understood Him.*
4   Made a searching and fearless moral inventory of ourselves.
5   Admitted to God, to ourselves, and to another human being the exact nature of our wrongs.
6   Were entirely ready to have God remove all these defects of character.
7   Humbly asked Him to remove our shortcomings.
8   Made a list of all persons we had harmed and became willing to make amends to them all.
9   Made direct amends to such people wherever possible, except when to do so would injure them or others.
10 Continued to take personal inventory and when we were wrong promptly admitted it.
11 Sought through prayer and meditation to improve our conscious contact with God *as we understood Him*, praying only for knowledge of His will for us and the power to carry that out.
12 Having had a spiritual awakening as the result of these steps, we tried to carry this message to alcoholics, and to practise these principles in all our affairs.

Note: The Twelve Steps are reprinted with permission of Alcoholics Anonymous World Services, Inc. Permission to reprint this material does not mean that AA has approved or reviewed the contents of this publication, nor that AA agrees with the views expressed herein. AA is a programme of recovery from alcoholism only – use of the Twelve Steps in connection with programmes and activities which are patterned after AA, but which address other problems, does not imply otherwise.

day at a time'. The aim is to concentrate on remaining abstinent for today and worry about tomorrow when it comes.

Therapeutic Communities

Therapeutic communities are residential programmes, often run by ex-addicts. A typical aim is to introduce structure into the life of the addict, and so there is emphasis on work and group activities. The new member begins with low status in terms of having few privileges and being allocated the most menial household chores. Change is encouraged by rewarding desired behaviour with increased status and privileges. Programmes are usually based upon the twelve-step programme, and include group therapy, individual counselling and education about drugs and alcohol. The central feature of many therapeutic communities is confrontation of the addict about his or her behaviour and attitudes by peers who 'have been there' (Kleber, 1989).

It was mentioned at the start of this chapter that levels of success in intervention are modest, yet much work is being done by academics and clinicians to improve this state of affairs. The quest for more effective interventions is important for those clients who are experiencing problems related to addiction; naturally, this to be applauded and supported. However, there is a parallel route that is also important – that of preventing problems arising in the first place. The next chapter deals with prevention.

Chapter 6

Prevention

The first question that must be asked in addressing the issue of prevention is what are we trying to prevent? Prevention may mean *inhibiting initiation* to substance use. Where smoking and illicit drug use are concerned, the preferred goal in many societies today is to eradicate these behaviours altogether, and one way to work towards this goal is to discourage people from taking them up in the first place. Prevention may also mean *inhibiting escalation* of substance use, that is encouraging people to keep to moderate, non-problematic levels. This is most clearly relevant to drinking alcohol; in western societies at least, prohibition is not the aim and therefore moderation is encouraged. Prevention can also include *inhibiting problems* associated with substance use. In cases where drinkers or drug users are unwilling or unable to reduce their consumption, priority may given to minimizing the adverse consequences associated with substance use.

Skirrow and Sawka (1987) base their ideas for alcohol and drug abuse prevention upon a number of assumptions, valid within western cultures. These assumptions are selectively summarized here. If we accept these assumptions, then we begin to see how prevention efforts should be directed. The first assumption is that levels of alcohol and drug-related problems are fundamentally related to the availability of alcohol and drugs, and to overall population consumption levels. If this is true, then it is important to *control the availability of alcohol and drugs*. The second assumption is that public support is necessary for the successful implementation of prevention programmes. Public support will depend upon a general acceptance that abstinence or moderation is best for the individual and for society, and also upon the knowledge that alternative opportunities are genuinely available for attaining the highest possible quality of life without recourse to alcohol or drugs. It follows from this that it is necessary to *change the culture and context in which drinking and drug use occur*. The third assumption is that drinking and drug use will never be eradicated in any society where the use of a given drug is accepted by a significant fraction of the population. If we accept this, then it is important to *provide individuals with the competencies to resist pressures to indulge or overindulge.* The fourth assumption is that the harmful consequences of the abuse of alcohol and drugs can be altered independent of actual levels of use. That is, action can be taken to minimize the severity of problems consequent upon drinking and drug use. This suggests that prevention programmes should also address *harm minimization.*

This chapter will be organized in four sections, based on the above assumptions: controls on availability; changing the culture and context; strengthening individual resilience; and harm minimization.

Controls on Availability

In Britain, as in other countries, the consensus view is that the use of alcohol and drugs is not a matter entirely for individual choice; that is, the rights of the individual are curtailed for the greater common good (Saunders, 1985). Where alcohol is concerned, there is legislation controlling availability by regulating who may manufacture alcohol for commercial purposes, who may sell it, how much it costs, who may purchase it, who may drink it, and when they may do so. The situation with regard to many drugs is one of prohibition. Laws exist to forbid the possession and use of certain drugs for non-medical purposes, and to ban the manufacture, sale and transportation of those drugs. These laws are applied most vigorously in interrupting the supply of drugs; reports regularly appear in the media about the apprehension of drug couriers by customs officials and the interruption of drug manufacture by police drug squads. More recently, the police have been petitioning the general public to assist by passing on information that will help them stamp out drugs.

At the simplest level, it may be stated that if a substance is not available to the individual, then consumption is not a possibility and consequently no problems will occur. The elimination of problematic substances, therefore, is the absolute solution. The reality, of course, is not that simple. We have seen already in Chapter 1 that prohibition of alcohol in the USA was not sustainable, primarily because it created an underground economy and a criminal subculture which the voting population was not willing to tolerate. Similar consequences may be observed as a by-product of the present 'war on drugs'.

Arguments for the benefits of introducing controls on the availability of alcohol are based on the premise that alcohol-related problems vary with overall per capita alcohol consumption in a population. That is, the more alcohol a population consumes, the greater will be the incidence of alcohol-related problems in that population. In 1956, a French researcher called Ledermann devised a formula by which one could, purportedly, calculate the incidence of heavy drinking based upon the knowledge of per capita alcohol consumption in any given population. Using this formula, it was demonstrated that any increase in the overall per capita alcohol consumption would lead to a higher proportion of the population falling into the heavy drinking category, the implication being that reducing alcohol consumption in the population as a whole would reduce the number of heavy drinkers. Ledermann's mathematics have since been discredited, leading some commentators to reject the entire notion that controls over alcohol are likely to lead to a reduction in alcohol-related damage. This may, however, be a case of throwing the baby out with the bath water; even though Ledermann's formula is incorrect, it is nevertheless true to say that per capita alcohol consumption is an indicator of a nation's health and well-being.

A commonly used indicator of harm is the level of liver cirrhosis mortality in a population. Those countries with high per capita alcohol consumption are also those with high levels of liver cirrhosis mortality. This may be demonstrated by comparing 'league tables' of alcohol consumption and cirrhosis mortality rates. For example, the Faculty of Public Health Medicine of the Royal College of Physicians (1991) report France, Portugal, Luxembourg, Spain, Italy, Hungary and western Germany as being amongst the top ten countries for both alcohol consumption and liver cirrhosis mortality. The use of liver cirrhosis as an indicator of harm has been criticized in that only a small number of drinkers die from liver cirrhosis, and others who do not drink excessively may also die from this condition. Saunders (1985) observes that, although the relationship between alcohol consumption and liver cirrhosis mortality is not one-to-one, there is a remarkable degree of concordance. In addition, cirrhosis mortality figures correlate with a wide range of disorders, including pancreatitis, cancers and circulatory diseases. Since cirrhosis co-varies with these disorders, the value of measuring cirrhosis mortality is therefore augmented.

It has often been suggested that alcohol consumption, and consequently liver cirrhosis, is highest in wine producing countries, where daily drinking is common, usually associated with meal times. In these cultures, regular steady drinking is the norm. By contrast, beer drinking is typical in north European countries and alcohol consumption occurs less frequently, being reserved for occasions where drinking is the main activity. Drinking in bouts is less likely to lead to physical damage, but is more likely to lead to intoxication and public disorder (Faculty of Public Health Medicine, The Royal College of Physicians, 1991).

Saunders (1985) points out that countries high in the alcohol consumption and liver cirrhosis mortality tables are typically those with fewer controls over the availability of alcohol. In support of the importance of the degree of control over alcohol, he cites the salutary experience of Finland, where controls changed over time and consequent problems reflected these changes. Between 1919 and 1932, alcohol was prohibited in Finland. After the repeal of prohibition, tight controls on the production and sale of alcohol were maintained by a state alcohol monopoly. The number of premises permitted to sell alcohol, the hours of sale, the type of beverage available, and the amount of alcohol purchasable on any one occasion were all strictly controlled. Citizens were also required to hold a certificate for the purchase of strong liquor, and these certificates could be withdrawn if alcohol-related laws were transgressed or if antisocial behaviour under the influence of alcohol was reported. In the late 1950s and throughout the 1960s, these controls over alcohol were relaxed. The number of liquor stores increased, opening hours were extended, purchase certificates were abolished, the legal drinking age was lowered, and the real price of alcohol was allowed to fall. The results of this liberalization were profound. Alcohol consumption rose dramatically, and so did deaths from liver cirrhosis, hospital admission rates for 'alcoholism', arrests for drunkenness, alcohol-related road traffic accidents and drunk-driving arrests. Since 1975, there has been a reversal toward restricting availability once again, and consumption levels have stabilized, as have the levels of alcohol-related problems.

The case for control seems, therefore, to be quite strong, and it is only the level of that control that remains open to public debate. What level of per capita consumption, and what level of alcohol-related problems, is society prepared to tolerate? Answers to these questions will inform decisions regarding the type and extent of controls instituted.

Control over the availability of alcohol is exercised in two major ways: licensing and taxation. The Faculty of Public Health Medicine of the Royal College of Physicians (1991) has issued recommendations for *licensing*. The first is that local licensing authorities should adopt clear policies for granting licences to sell alcohol. While some licensing issues are determined by national government (e.g. the lower age limit for purchasing alcohol), other issues are controlled locally. Granting licences to sell alcohol has implications for the community in terms of public safety, public nuisance, likelihood of non-compliance with the law and local levels of alcohol abuse. If licensing practices are to contribute to problem prevention, then the implications of granting licences and ways of responding to licence applications should be thoroughly considered and set forth in an explicit policy. A second recommendation is that every police authority should have a written statement of intent regarding surveillance of licensed premises and preventive policing of those areas identifiable as likely to give rise to alcohol-related problems. Clearly, there is no point in having licensing restrictions if these cannot be enforced, and information on this could be taken into account by local licensing authorities in making decisions about who should be granted a licence to sell alcohol.

Where *taxation* is concerned, one economics axiom is that demand is determined by price relative to income, and so it is possible to manipulate the demand for alcohol by adjusting taxation levels (Maynard, 1985). Overall levels of taxation can be adjusted, but also duties on alcohol can be banded to reflect the alcohol content of a drink so that the higher the alcohol content, the more expensive the drink. However, the government is guided by a number of different objectives when determining taxation levels, including generating revenue, fostering employment and controlling inflation. It is not difficult to see how these objectives may conflict with each other, and how limiting alcohol consumption through increases in taxation may, in fact, kill the goose that lays the golden egg (Maynard, 1985). The Faculty of Public Health Medicine of the Royal College of Physicians (1991) recommends that the government should adopt a taxation policy that explicitly states that the aim is to reduce alcohol consumption. One criticism of restrictions by way of price increases is that this will not deter the heavy drinker, but merely impinge upon the freedoms of the moderate drinker. Heavy drinkers, it is argued, will simply change to cheaper drinks, or switch their spending from necessities to alcohol, perhaps to the detriment of themselves and their families. Saunders (1985) challenges this criticism by presenting evidence that price increases curtail drinking in *all* drinkers, heavy or otherwise. In any case, it can be argued that reducing consumption amongst moderate drinkers is no bad thing in respect of a nation's health.

While there appears to be a case for tightening controls over the availability of alcohol, the opposite could be argued with regard to illicit drugs. A number of commentators have observed that drug prohibition laws incur certain financial and social costs. Nadelmann

(1988) identifies a number of these costs. There is the financial burden to the tax payer of expenditure on law enforcement, including paying customs officials and the police, financing the legal processing of offenders through the courts, and bearing the costs of imprisonment of offenders. He points out that there is also a hidden cost here in that targeting drug offenders necessarily means that resources are not directed towards other types of crime. Drug laws also create a criminal subculture. Drug dealers can make vast profits from their activities, and they are often prepared to protect their market by violent methods. As Nadelmann (1988) says of the US situation, 'In many neighborhoods, it often seems to be the aggressive, gun-toting drug dealers who upset residents far more than addicts nodding in doorways' (p. 101). The individual drug user is also forced into criminality, first by being labelled a criminal by virtue of drug use alone, and second through having to resort to criminal activities to purchase drugs at inflated street prices. Finally, the illicit nature of drug use creates risks for the individual. Forcing people into the position of having to share needles is one obvious concern, given the risk of HIV infection. In addition, the illicit market does not exercise quality control, and there are risks from using unexpectedly potent or adulterated drugs.

Nadelmann (1988) suggests that it is necessary to examine the situation rationally, and to distinguish between the problems of drug use and the problems that result from prohibition policies. The moral justification of drug prohibition is to protect those who, if drugs were available, would use these drugs and cause harm to themselves or others. Nadelmann says,

> But ultimately the moral quality of laws must be judged not by how those laws are intended to work in principle, but how they function in fact. When laws intended to reflect a moral obligation cause new harms of a different kind, arguably even greater in impact, there is a need to re-evaluate them and inquire whether those laws have become in some sense immoral. (p. 97)

Nadelmann (1988) presents a case for drug legalization: the tax payer would be relieved of bearing the costs of law enforcement; pressure within the criminal justice system would be reduced; and drug dealers would be put out of business. Set prices would mean that drug users would have less need to resort to crime to support their habit, and the introduction of quality controls and government health education would ensure that drug users are better informed about the substance they are using. In addition to the reduction of these problems, state control of the drug market would mean the introduction of taxes and duties, contributing to the nation's economy.

One common assumption, which leads to resistance to the notion of change, is that legalization means a free market and unrestricted availability of drugs for all. Nadelmann (1992) points out that the options are not simply either drug prohibition or no controls whatsoever, but rather that drug control policies lie along a continuum between these two polar opposites. Both the prohibitionists and those on the side of drug legalization have more in common than might at first appear. Their aims are similar in that both groups want to minimize drug-related problems; it is simply that their proposed strategies differ. Where prohibitionists rely heavily on the criminal justice system to control drugs, those who favour legalization would wish to emphasize a public health approach. However, legal regulation of the manufacture and sale of drugs is obviously necessary, just as many other substances are controlled to varying degrees, for example alcohol, tobacco and prescribed drugs. The point is not to abandon all limits, but simply to review the situation with regard to illicit drugs rationally and dispassionately.

Nadelmann (1992) points out that

> Few drug control regimes are static. Prohibitions, regulations, and decriminalizations tend to evolve as new drugs emerge, as drug use patterns shift, as other drug-related norms change, and as popular and élite perceptions of various drugs, drug consumers, and drug problems shift. (p. 114)

What policy makers ought to address are the *best* means of regulating the production, distribution and consumption of drugs, through an objective and systematic evaluation of the costs and benefits of various policy options. Since much of the damage caused by illicit drugs is a consequence of prohibition policies, either through criminal activities or forcing people into the position of consuming drugs in dangerous ways, legalization, argues Nadelmann (1989), 'affords far greater opportunities to control drug use and abuse than do current criminalization policies' (p. 945). Nadelmann (1988) concludes that, while there can be no guarantee that legalization, even with controls on availability, would lead to a reduction in drug use, it is almost certain that the financial and social costs of current drug prohibition policies would be reduced.

The arguments presented above suggest that controls over alcohol need to be tightened and that controls over drugs might advantageously be loosened. Marks (1991) says that 'In order to control the supply of drugs or alcohol, it would appear the state must provide a (legal) supply. For control is lost if supply is too lax (as with alcohol) or so restricted that the available sources are criminal (as with heroin)' (p. 314).

Changing the Culture and Context

When referring to the environment in which substance use occurs, this may be taken to include both the social milieu, including prevailing social norms, and the structural context, including the characteristics of those settings in which substance use may occur and the availability of opportunities for alternative activities.

It has been argued that

> even in the absence of formal legal controls, informal social control and self-control factors would prevent most people from serious drug involvement. If so, then a change in drug laws might open some spigots, but it would not open any floodgates. Most current non-users would remain non-users. (MacCoun, 1993, p. 507)

This statement suggests that informal factors play a major role in controlling substance use, and perhaps a greater role than legal sanctions.

Social norms may be defined as 'the implicit rules and expectations that dictate what we ought to think and how we ought to behave' (Atkinson *et al.*, 1993, p. 749). Social norms operate to determine an individual's behaviour in two stages. First, the individual observes how a reference group behaves, and conducts himself or herself according to what is perceived as acceptable in any situation. Of course, there are numerous reference groups for each individual, including family, peers and authority figures. Norms vary from one group to the next, and their impact on the individual will vary depending upon the degree of bonding to any particular group and the specific social context at the time, for example whether one is at home with the family or out with friends. Second, the individual's behaviour is instrumentally conditioned to conform to social norms. Behaviour that is consistent with social norms is reinforced by approval and acceptance, and behaviour that is inconsistent with social norms is punished by disapproval, ridicule and rejection (MacCoun, 1993).

One way of controlling substance use, then, is to change social norms so that they become less favourable towards substance use. This has been tackled mainly through *health education*. Educational approaches are based on the notion that, if a person knows the facts about alcohol and drugs, then the rational choice will be to avoid their use altogether or at least to avoid excessive use.

The obvious place to start alcohol and drug education is in schools. Stuart (1974) investigated the effects of alcohol and drug education on junior high school students. The programme included information about the pharmacology of alcohol and drugs and their physiological effects. Comparing students in the education group with a no-education control group, Stuart found that the education group showed a significant increase in knowledge about alcohol and drugs, yet at the same time they also showed significantly *greater* levels of self-reported alcohol and drug use.

In a review of school alcohol and drug education programmes by Kinder *et al.* (1980), education was shown consistently to increase knowledge, but also to exacerbate rather than reduce alcohol and drug use. Hopkins *et al.* (1988) conducted a comprehensive evaluation of a large scale alcohol education programme in American schools. This programme was designed to

1   increase students' knowledge about alcohol and its effects;
2   encourage attitudes favouring abstinence or moderation;
3   enhance self-esteem; and
4   teach skills for responsible decision making regarding alcohol use.

Data were collected over three years from almost 7000 students, of whom around 4000 had undertaken the programme and 3000 had not. Again, the effect of education was to increase knowledge, but there was no impact at all on drinking behaviour. Hopkins *et al.* concluded that the educational programme simply 'did not work' (p. 48).

Despite the prevalent view that alcohol and drug education is a worthwhile pursuit, research tells us that this approach is at best ineffective, and may in some cases even be counterproductive in that it increases substance use. Given the amount of time and effort devoted to education, there is an obvious need to look closely at why programmes do not work and see if anything can be done to make education more effective.

One possibility is that alcohol and drug education programmes are not targeted at the people who need them. In schools, such programmes are often part of the general curriculum, thus they include pupils who are *not* likely to go on to drink excessively or to use drugs. This group could be adversely affected by education through labelling; that is, since they have been included in the programme, they may assume that they are seen to be at risk for problem drinking or drug use, and this may become a self-fulfilling prophecy. Alternatively, education may give rise to a curiosity factor, where young people test out the truth of what they have been told by drinking or using drugs when they had not previously intended to do so.

A second possibility is that alcohol and drug education programmes may contain information that is inappropriate for young people. Where the content of such programmes centres around the long term serious health consequences of substance use, young people often cannot relate this information to their own experience. At this stage in psychological development, the consideration of one's own mortality is not a big issue, and it is also probable that most substance users of young people's acquaintance suffer no apparent health problems. In relation to drinking, for example, to emphasize the risks of liver cirrhosis, brain damage and cancers may simply convey the message that only 'alcoholics' need concern themselves about their drinking, and that the majority of drinkers (themselves included) have no cause for worry.

It is also true that 'scare tactics' have generally been shown to be ineffective in changing behaviour. One reason for this is that raising anxiety about the consequences of substance use can be so uncomfortable for the individual that anxiety reduction becomes the most urgent concern, and this may be achieved in ways other than behaviour change, for example by avoiding exposure to further information or by thinking that 'it won't happen to me'. A specific example of this is where pictures of blackened lungs are shown to smokers in an attempt to scare them out of their habit. This raises anxiety to the extent that many smokers block out consideration of the possible consequences – they simply do not bear thinking about. Ironically, for those whose main reason for using drink or drugs is as a means of reducing anxiety, there is always the risk that scare tactics will actually increase their substance use.

The content of alcohol and drug education programmes should be appropriate, but so too should be the way that the message is conveyed. Some useful information about both content and style of presentation comes from studies of 'psychological reactance' to alcohol education with college students. Reactance is the term used to describe a response in a situation involving a threat to freedom that is directed towards re-establishing that freedom. Bensley and Wu (1991) gave two types of alcohol education to college students. The first was 'high threat' and contained dogmatic phrases such as 'any reasonable person must acknowledge the conclusions'; the second was 'low threat' and contained neutral phrases such as 'we believe that these conclusions are reasonable'. Half of the students were given the high threat message, and half were given the low threat message. Each group was further subdivided so that half were advised to abstain from alcohol and half were advised to keep to moderate drinking levels. In their first study, Bensley and Wu (1991) asked subjects about their intentions regarding future drinking and found that the high threat message, particularly when combined with an abstinence recommendation, resulted in more intentions to drink. Overall, heavier drinkers showed a greater reactance effect. Bensley and Wu carried their study one step further with a different group of subjects using a measure of actual drinking. Under the guise of a supposed taste test of different beers, the researchers monitored how much people drank following high and low threat education. Of all their student subjects – male and female, heavy and moderate drinkers, those who received high threat and those who received low threat messages – they found that male students who were heavy drinkers and had received the high threat message drank most. These studies indicate that a dogmatic approach to alcohol education, especially when combined with an abstinence recommendation, can be counterproductive, especially for male heavy drinkers. The lesson from this is that alcohol education should be presented in a non-threatening manner and provide guidelines for sensible drinking rather than commands to abstain.

A third possible explanation for the ineffectiveness of education is that it may be futile without accompanying skills training. That is, it is not sufficient to advise people to be abstinent or moderate without teaching them how to go about it. Interesting findings have come from studies using the statistical technique of meta-analysis, where outcome measures from a large number of well-designed studies can be summarized and analysed to answer the question 'What works?' A meta-analysis of smoking and alcohol use prevention programmes revealed that the least effective programmes are those based on traditional awareness-raising, and the more successful programmes are those that teach people how cope with the pressures to smoke and drink (Rundall and Bruvold, 1988). Similarly, a meta-analysis of drug use prevention programmes showed that those that focused upon helping young people to resist peer pressure, improve their communication skills, and build up feelings of competence were far superior to those that attempted simply to increase knowledge about drugs or change attitudes to them (Tobler, 1986). It is interesting to note that 'peer counsellors' may be the best people for the job of skills training. Since peer pressure is an important influence in adolescent drinking and drug use, it has been suggested that peer pressure could be used positively by training adolescents to become counsellors to their peers (Swadi and Zeitlin, 1988).

Moving on from school-based education programmes to mass media communication, it becomes apparent that many similar issues pertain. The media – television, radio, newspapers, magazines and posters – have become important channels of communication in society. If the intended message is to be conveyed effectively, then it is necessary to know how mass media communication works. Wilde (1993) identifies a number of key components in effective media communication. First, the message is likely to be more influential if the receiver considers the *conveyor* to have high levels of credibility, expertise and trustworthiness, and a perceived similarity with the receiver. Second, there are a number of important issues relating to the *message.* This should be within a latitude of acceptability; that is it should contain some views already held by the receiver, yet also advocate change, but not too much change. The message should be personally relevant, contain concrete instructions rather then general slogans (e.g. Just Say No!), avoid a paternalistic manner, and model the target behaviour. The message should also catch one's attention, and have a motivating appeal by bearing relevance to what people are trying to achieve (e.g. prestige, or a sense of belonging). Third, the *channel of communication* is important in that the choice of channel should take into account the exposure rate in the particular group at whom the message is targeted, and there should be an immediacy factor whereby the message should be received when and where the behaviour is actually occurring.

Clearly, this knowledge about how mass media communication works may be used both for promoting substance use, as in advertising, and for promoting abstinence or moderation, as in health education. In his review, Wilde (1993) suggests that many studies are conducted to assess the effectiveness of advertising, but that much of this knowledge remains confidential. On the other hand, very little research is conducted to examine the effectiveness of health education. The evidence relating to bans on advertising is equivocal; some studies have shown that bans decrease substance use, but others have shown no effect. Wilde (1993) cites one study which showed that a 'fairness doctrine' was effective in reducing cigarette consumption in the USA. Here, cigarette advertisements were not banned, but broadcasters had to allocate an equal amount of air time to antismoking messages. Wilde comments that this fits in well with the concept of agenda-setting, which holds that the media are powerful in their ability to influence what the people *think about*, rather than what they *think*. Wilde (1993) suggests that

> presentation of the various sides of an issue in the mass media can be expected to increase the personally experienced salience of health-related decisions such as to smoke or not to smoke, to drink or not to drink, and what drinking in moderation means . . . Because of the fact that people do not passively absorb the content of mass communications and do not simply act according to the content printed or broadcast, mass media information should not be considered equivalent to mass indoctrination (p. 992).

None of this is to say that advertising practices should not be controlled. The features of successful mass communication presented earlier suggest that alcohol and cigarettes should not be endorsed by certain kinds of people, for example media figures with whom the viewing population can closely identify, such as popular soap opera characters. Motivation to drink or smoke should not be encouraged through assertions that consumption will enhance a person's sexual prowess, physical capabilities or social desirability. Sponsorship of sports personalities and sporting events by cigarette or alcohol manufacturers is obviously anomalous here, since this implies at least that smoking and drinking are not disadvantageous to physical fitness. Advertising should not be aimed at persuading non-users, particularly young people, to take up drinking or smoking or persuading existing drinkers and smokers to consume more. The situation at present is that codes of advertising, some legal and some voluntary, do in fact impose such restrictions.

A great deal of money is spent on advertising tobacco and alcohol compared with the amount spent on health education. Despite limited resources, health education in the media should be designed for maximum effectiveness. Past attempts have helped identify where it is possible to go wrong with the design of media health education. Thorley (1985) reports on a media campaign staged in the northeast of England in the 1970s. This was run by the Health Education Council, with the media programme designed by an advertising company, and evaluation conducted by a market research firm. The aims were to publicize the dangers of heavy drinking, educate the public to recognize the signs of problems, and tell people where to get help. No significant changes in drinking behaviour in the area were apparent. Thorley suggests that one of the reasons for failure was that the messages were vague and inappropriate. For example, the instruction to 'drink sensibly' was found to be unhelpful since there was no advice about what 'sensible' means. In fact, as the campaign progressed, more specific advice was given – two or three pints, two or three times a week – and this was better received.

Attention obviously needs to be paid to the message conveyed in media health campaigns. Messages should be targeted at specific sectors of the population, using media channels that will reach them. Young people form one important target group. Media messages should be delivered by credible people with whom the target group can identify, and should motivate people by advising them of the advantages of abstinence or moderation and the disadvantages of excessive consumption. This is akin to a motivational interviewing style, in that acknowledging the positive aspects of substance use leads people on to consideration of the negative aspects (O'Connor, 1990). The information should be personally and immediately relevant. With young people, for example, health is not usually the most important or immediate concern. It is interesting to note that one antismoking campaign which, anecdotally at least, appeared particularly influential with young people was one in which a picture of an attractive teenager smoking a cigarette was matched with the message 'It's like kissing an ashtray'. Young people are usually more immediately concerned about what the boyfriend or girlfriend thinks than they are about the long term possibilities of emphysema, heart disease and lung cancer.

Thorley (1985) points out that the media campaign in the northeast of England had some positive 'side effects', such as a media interest in alcohol issues – 'booze is news'. Prime-time television programmes about alcohol were produced, and newspapers ran articles about alcohol issues, which constituted a free media campaign. The campaign fell short of its ideals by failing to provide adequate back-up services in the community. The agencies advertised as offering help were deluged with enquiries and could not meet the demand, which was something of an embarrassment. As a consequence of this, there was a development of community services for drinkers. Furthermore, many employers asked for advice about work place alcohol policies. Obviously, these 'side effects' are not to be dismissed; media campaigns should be seen as long term strategies that take effect in a variety of different ways.

It may be wise, however, for health educators to acknowledge that, while information may be provided, it is also useful to nudge people in the right direction by limiting their behaviour. Operating upon the premise that knowledge changes attitudes that in turn change behaviour may, in fact, be less effective than working the other way round – change behaviour first, and a change in attitudes will follow. One potent example of changing the culture and context these days relates to smoking. It is becoming increasingly common for smoking to be prohibited in public places, such as on public transport, in offices, in cinemas and in some restaurants. One further place where rules about substance use may be set and relatively easily enforced is in the work place.

Work place policies have arisen as a consequence of the realization that addictive behaviours can cause problems at work that are costly for employers. Absenteeism owing to ailments related to drinking and smoking, impaired efficiency and increased likelihood of accidents all have adverse economic consequences. Where smoking is concerned, action may be taken against an employer by a non-smoker whose health has been damaged as a result of 'passive smoking', that is exposure to environmental tobacco smoke (Howard, 1990). These issues have undoubtedly prompted many employers to consider their stance regarding drinking and smoking by the work force.

Tether and Robinson (1986) suggest that a comprehensive alcohol policy should define the rules for inappropriate drinking, and provide back-up support for identified problem drinkers. Inappropriate drinking includes drinking at work and coming to work under the influence of alcohol. A clear statement of rules regarding drinking and disciplinary procedures for breach of these rules should be made. However, in discouraging drinking at work, employers have a responsibility to consider the work environment. A work place bar, wine produced at lunchtime meetings, and discounts offered on the sale of alcohol to employees may all encourage drinking, and inadequate canteen facilities may drive people to local pubs at meal times. Changes may, therefore, need to be made to the context in addition to setting rules for behaviour.

The second component of a good work place alcohol policy is to provide help and support for the employee identified as having a problem with alcohol. Firing that person obviously solves the problem in one way, but this is a costly option in that recruitment and training new staff to do the job are expensive procedures. Supervisors, managers and personnel staff should be trained to identify staff with a drinking problem. Typical signs are absenteeism, particularly on a Monday morning, inefficiency, accidents and decreased ability to get along with work colleagues. Once identified, the employee should be offered help, either from internal services such as an occupational health nurse, or through contact with a community service, such as a local Council on Alcohol.

Smoking policies follow similar lines. In many work places, smoking is banned in communal areas, such as open plan offices, meeting rooms and canteens. Some organizations ban smoking in all indoor areas, but many provide a room where smoking is permitted. Help for those who wish to quit smoking is available in some organizations. Klesges *et al.* (1987) report the use of self-help reading materials and advice from a physician, both of which have only modest success in reducing smoking, but are low cost procedures which can be administered widely. Behavioural group interventions show better outcome, but are more expensive to run and cannot always be offered to the entire work force. Incentive-based programmes appear to be most promising in terms of cost-effectiveness. Here, financial incentives are given to employees who abstain from smoking. In some cases, incentives may be awarded to teams who show best progress, thus encouraging non-smokers to exert influence over their smoker colleagues.

It is obvious that if people are to be successfully dissuaded from drinking and drug use, appealing *alternatives* need to be available to them. Tobler (1986), in her meta-analysis of drug use prevention programmes, found that directing adolescents into more positive activities was effective, particularly for specific subgroups who were already abusers or who were presenting problems at school. The types of alternative activities included in these programmes were finding jobs, doing voluntary work, attendance at youth clubs, sport and reading. Where a young person has not had access to opportunities such as these, it can help to facilitate their development.

Yates and Hebblethwaite (1985) suggest that prevention should capitalize upon naturally occurring methods for curtailing drinking. They ask what events in the ordinary life of a community influence people to refrain from drinking too much? The availability of other entertainments and activities is one diversion from drinking. If there is something else that appeals, then people are less likely to wish to drink to excess and so miss out on other opportunities.

Strengthening Individual Resilience

One way of looking at prevention is in terms of attenuating those factors which present a risk for substance use and associated problems, and strengthening those factors that protect against substance use and associated problems. Each individual is exposed to different risk factors and has different personal qualities to protect him or her in the face of those risk factors. Prevention efforts aim to *decrease vulnerability*, that is to minimize risk factors, and to *increase resilience*, that is to enhance protective factors.

In their investigation of factors associated with adolescent substance use, Kumpfer and Turner (1990) found that mixing with antisocial (i.e. nonconforming or delinquent) peers was the most influential factor. However, whether young people chose to associate with antisocial or prosocial peers was influenced by degrees of school bonding and levels of personal self-esteem. These factors were, in turn, influenced by family and school climate; poor family or school climate inhibits the development of school bonding and a positive self-image. Kumpfer and Turner (1990) use this information to suggest how prevention programmes might be effectively developed. The 'new breed' of prevention programmes should aim to improve family and school environments, as well as aiming to teach skills for coping with peer pressure to drink or use drugs.

Oetting (1992) represents this comprehensive psychosocial model of prevention as a wheel (see Figure 6.1). The child is at the hub of the wheel and is connected to the three primary socialization contexts of family, school and peer groups through the spokes of the wheel. Each of these major socialization contexts needs to be 'healthy' in terms of promoting prosocial behaviours in the child, and the links between the child and its family, school and peers need to be strong. The rim of the wheel represents bonds between family, school and peers. When all of these areas are strongly bonded together, the wheel is robust and the chances of deviant behaviour, including drinking and drug use are reduced. A number of interventions to strengthen the 'wheel' have been developed.

Family

Family support programmes enable risk factors to be addressed when children are young, well before initiation to substance use. Family factors that place a young person at risk for drinking and drug use were described in Chapter 3, and include poor family management practices, low bonding to parents and high levels of family conflict. Clearly, poor monitoring and control of behaviour creates the circumstances whereby the young person is at liberty to engage in drinking, drug use, delinquency and the like. Indeed, family management is implicated in the

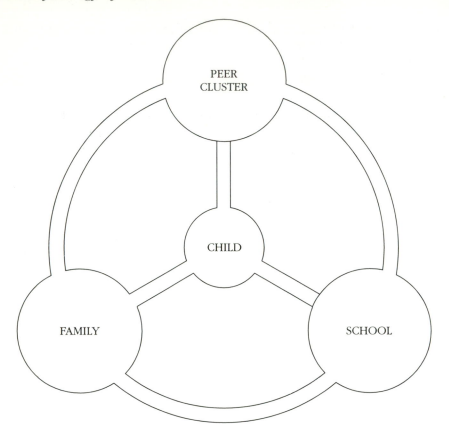

Figure 6.1   *A model for prevention of deviant behaviour*
Note: *Copyright 1991 – E.R. Oetting, Tri-Ethnic Center for Prevention Research, Fort Collins, CO. Reproduced with permission.*

cluster of problem behaviours identified by Jessor and Jessor (1977) in their problem behaviour theory (see Chapter 2). When a child engages in these problem behaviours, this may prove stressful for the family, and it may well be that members of such a family escape the stress through alcohol or drug use. Young family members are then at risk of learning to use substances to help them cope with problems since this is modelled by their parents. Obviously, these issues need to be addressed in family support programmes.

Hawkins *et al.* (1992), in their review of family support programmes, summarize the effective components of interventions with parents. Parents should be taught the skills to

(a)   set clear expectations for behavior,
(b)   monitor and supervise their children,

(c)   consistently reinforce prosocial behavior,

(d)   create opportunities for family involvement, and

(e)   promote the development of their children's academic, social and refusal skills. (p. 93)

Family support programmes have been shown to influence delinquency and academic performance as well as substance use (Hawkins *et al.*, 1992).

Herbert (1987) suggests that family work should be conducted in the home, since behaviour is best viewed as a function of the total environment, and that the aim should be to teach parents the principles of behaviour change. He describes the 'triadic' model of intervention, the triad being the professional, the parent or caretaker, and the child. The professional visits the home of the family that has requested assistance and begins an assessment of the problem. After a thorough assessment, a programme for change is designed and the child's parents or caretakers are trained and supported in implementing this change programme. The professional acts as a consultant to the family, so that the parents can learn strategies for controlling the child's behaviour. These may then be used consistently by the parents in the natural environment, thus providing a long term solution to the problem.

School

The child's degree of involvement with school may prevent substance use by encouraging attachment to prosocial peers and engagement in prosocial activities. Interventions aimed at changing teaching practices, classroom management and school organization are important here. Cooperative learning approaches have shown positive effects upon attitudes to school, bonding with prosocial peers and academic achievement. Here, children of differing abilities work together as a team, thus encouraging them to help and support others. This approach holds promise for reducing risk for substance use and requires further investigation (Hawkins *et al.*, 1992). Kumpfer and Turner (1990) outline their comprehensive approach to creating a positive school environment. This includes cooperative learning, peer counselling, faculty retreats, school pride days and class support activities. They predict that the effects of such programmes will take some time to show, since changing the school climate is not something that can be achieved overnight.

Peers

Where peer groups are concerned, Elliott *et al.* (1985) point out that interventions to alter peer friendship networks are not common. In fact, many intervention programmes actually facilitate the development of antisocial peer groups, in that they gather together drinkers, drug users or delinquents. When such a group is gathered together, it is unreasonable to expect that they will generate a prosocial set of values. Elliott *et al.* (1985) emphasize that efforts should be made to integrate high risk youth into conventional peer groups. They suggest that parents should monitor their children's friends, that at-risk youth should be dispersed across schools and classes rather than be grouped together, and that attempts should be made to bond children with prosocial groups. This last suggestion indicates that encouraging children to attend church, Scouts and activity groups could be beneficial, and the community should provide such opportunities if it wishes to promote prosocial behaviours.

Children

The child is at the centre of Oetting's 'wheel', and children who are at risk of developing substance use problems may require individual attention. Oetting (1992) suggests that some children 'may have traits that make bonding difficult or that interfere with communication of appropriate norms' (p. 335). He gives examples of two such characteristics – anger and sensation-seeking. Oetting says that anger may damage bonds with the family and school, thus setting the scene for association with deviant peer groups. Clearly, anger management training would be helpful in building closer bonds with the family and school, although more direct steps towards building better relationships would also be required. Where sensation seeking is concerned, this is not in itself a bad thing; the problem lies in channelling the young person's energies into socially acceptable goals. Indeed, part of the rationale behind outdoor activity programmes is to show that excitement can be found

Table 6.1 *Prevention programme (Rhodes and Jason, 1988)*

1 *Understanding adolescence*
  Discussion of physical and emotional changes.
2 *Skills for life*
  Identification of the skills required for adult life.
3 *Self-Esteem*
  How to feel good about yourself and how to make others feel good about themselves.
4 *Communication skills*
  Listening to others and expressing your feelings.
5 *Decision making*
  How to stop and think through a problem in order to come to a decision.
6 *Substances*
  Information about drink, drugs and cigarettes.
7 *Identifying pressures to use drugs*
  Looking at the messages about substances conveyed through the media, advertisements, peer pressure and adult modelling.
8 *Resisting peer pressure*
  Assertiveness and refusal skills training; Saying 'No thanks' to substances.
9 *Goal setting*
  Identifying short and longer term goals in life.

through canoeing, abseiling and other such pursuits instead of drinking, drug use or delinquency.

Since substance use is strongly predicted by association with substance using peers, it seems important to arm young people with the skills for resisting peer pressure. Considerable emphasis has been placed upon teaching children and adolescents assertiveness skills and refusal skills. Kumpfer and Turner (1990) take issue with this simplistic approach by asking what exactly is meant by 'peer pressure'. Often, this is understood to be a direct badgering by friends along the lines of 'Go on, have a drink – don't be a wimp'. While this sort of peer pressure may be exerted upon young people, indirect pressure could be more influential. Indirect pressure manifests itself in feeling the need to be part of the group, that is not wanting to be left out when others are drinking or using drugs. Most prevention programmes these days address a range of elements, as exemplified by that of Rhodes and Jason (1988) that is outlined in Table 6.1.

May (1993), however, recognizes that 'the definition of adolescents who misuse alcohol as socially incompetent individuals, unable to resist contamination by group influences is misplaced' (p. 163). He suggests that it may be more useful to turn attention back to substances as the problem rather than to view the consumer as the problem. In doing this, it becomes logical to teach young people how to consume substances safely. This leads on to broader issues of harm minimization.

Harm Minimization

McKechnie (1985) suggests that to talk of 'alcohol-related problems' focuses attention upon alcohol and directs efforts to reduce those problems at reducing alcohol consumption. If, however, these problems are viewed as related to the context in which they occur, then it becomes apparent that there are other measures which may be taken to reduce harm. That is, in addition to reducing drinking *per se*, direct action may be taken to minimize the problems consequent upon drinking. Reducing the negative consequences of drinking for the drinker is sometimes resisted on the grounds that, by doing so, one is removing the need to change levels of alcohol consumption. Tober (1991) suggests that this resistance is based upon two false assumptions: that greater suffering will always lead to a reduction in drinking, and that a reduction in drinking will result only from increased suffering. She points out that, while greater suffering can lead to a reduction in drinking, it can also lead to increased drinking to relieve that suffering. In addition, many people reduce their drinking for positive reasons, such as finding a new job, a new love or new interests in life. Whether drinking is reduced to avoid suffering or better to enjoy the positive aspects of life, it is preferable that, when the new day dawns, the drinker has sustained as little damage as possible.

One problem that society would wish to reduce is road traffic accidents. While continuing to persuade people not to drink and drive, at the same time other action may be taken. One example of a change to the environment aimed at minimizing harm is to make cars more robust so that if an accident should occur, then the occupants of the car are less likely to be hurt. Making roads safer for drivers and pedestrians is another option, for example by better lighting, which would reduce the likelihood of accidents, and erecting crash barriers, which would minimize damage if an accident did occur. It is also possible to make starting a car more complex, for example by making ignition of the engine dependent upon carrying out some operation within a set time limit. Drivers impaired by alcohol would find themselves less likely to be able to get the car going. While none of these measures gives complete protection against alcohol-related road traffic accidents, they do offer some measure of harm minimization, and they also offer a general contribution to road safety.

Town planning is another fertile area for making changes that limit harm. Alcohol-related crime, particularly offences of violence, typically occurs in and around city centre pubs and clubs after closing time

(Hope, 1985; Ramsay, 1982). Hope (1985) comments that city centres in Britain are nowadays primarily designed to service those who come into the city by day. Pedestrian precincts, underground walkways, and multi-storey car parks benefit workers and shoppers, but, in the absence of a residential population to care for the area, a city centre can become an indefensible public space late at night. He suggests that attention should be paid to urban planning and design in order to avoid such problems. Other strategies to reduce alcohol-related violence are staggering closing times of licensed premises to avoid having the entire drinking population decanted into the streets at the same time; facilitating the dispersal of people from the city centre by improving public transport; altering the character of pubs and clubs so that disorder becomes less likely; and teaching bar staff the management techniques and interpersonal skills for minimizing risk (Hope, 1985).

Training the managers and staff of licensed premises is common in Canada. This has its basis in the emergence of civil liability, that is where providers of alcohol may be held liable for damages or injuries caused by intoxicated customers or guests (Single, 1993). Single cites the tale of a club patron known only as 'Sunshine' who climbed onto a roof support beam to 'moon' at the other customers. Sunshine fell on one unfortunate man, who later took action against the club for allowing unsafe activities on the premises. This incident has its amusing side, but many accidents and fights have consequences which are no joke. One response in Canada, therefore, has been to introduce training for bartenders and managers. Programmes include information about alcohol and the law, and alcohol and health. Staff are also trained how to recognize intoxication and deal with drunk customers. Research evidence suggests that these programmes successfully reduce intoxication without adverse effects on profit. Extra takings from the sale of food and non-alcoholic beverages off-set the loss of sales to drunk customers, and there are savings from lower insurance premiums against civil liability (Single, 1993).

Problem prevention may also involve families. Tober (1991) suggests that partners of problem drinkers may be assisted in taking practical steps to minimize harm, such as protecting the family income, guarding against accidents in the home, and ensuring that children are able to cope with crises (for example, by telephoning a responsible adult). She also points out that families should 'reject the drinking and not the drinker' (Tober, 1991, p. 31). Expressing anger and disapproval when a partner is intoxicated, pouring drink away, and refusing to have alcohol in the house are all rejections of drinking behaviour. By

owing to the association between drug use and HIV transmission. The prevention of HIV infection has now become a priority. Consequently, there has been a shift away from looking at issues of addiction and characteristics of the drug user; nowadays, the focus is on the specific behaviour of drug injection. Stimson (1990) says, 'Rather than seeing drug use as a metaphorical disease, there is now a real medical problem associated with injecting drugs' (p. 333). Stimson's remark should remind us of Chapter 1, in which attitudes to drinking and drug use in the seventeenth and eighteenth centuries were described. In those days, drinking and drug use were not viewed as problems in themselves, but problems *related* to drinking and drug use were acknowledged. It seems, then, that the addictions wheel may have turned a full circle.

If society is to cope with the problems associated with substance use, then it is imperative that we should take a wide view of the relevant issues. Davies (1992) recommends

> a more systems-based approach, within which inputs from drug users and treatment specialists play a role as a necessary and essential part, but which accords equal status to historical and geographical factors, to political and government agendas, to the role of newspapers and television, the broader social and political climate within which drug use takes place, up to and including everyone living within that social system, and the attitudes and values they learn, and which they bring to the issue. (p. 164)

Psychologists should not consider themselves exempt from this advice; they should look beyond the individual in their search for explanations of addictive behaviours and effective interventions for preventing and ameliorating problems related to substance use.

Individual therapy is only one amongst a range of strategies for dealing with addictive behaviours and the problems associated with them, yet it has its place. Therapeutic approaches must, however, move with the times. Davies (1992) points out that harm minimization requires that we view drug users as responsible for and in control over their substance use:

> People believing themselves to be helpless cannot guide or take responsibility for their actions; and the involvement of HIV with drug use now requires with some urgency that drug users do exactly that . . . The link between HIV and IV [intravenous] drug use now makes it imperative that if people decide to use

drugs, and many people make that decision and will continue to do so, then they should use their drugs competently above all else. (p. 161)

Where interventions with individual substance users are concerned, the range of goals needs to be widened to include safer practices, as well as reducing levels of drinking and drug use. Furthermore, the approaches used should be those that increase the client's feelings of self-efficacy. As Peele (1985) says, 'Therapy works best when it requires clients to change attitudes, practise skills, and make life changes and when it attributes these changes to the client' (p. 144). This is consistent with giving responsibility back to the individual while remaining helpful and encouraging.

Clearly, many advances in the study of addictive behaviours have been made over the years, yet the context in which our knowledge may be put to use is continually changing. There is, and will continue to be, a need for further debate, research and development in clinical practice. Perhaps those stalwart readers who have reached the end of this book will enter active service.

Chapter 7

Postscript

Having read this far, some readers may wish for further information or advice about alcohol or drugs. First of all, it would be improper to conclude this book without giving some direction to those readers who may wish to seek help with their own drinking or drug use. In most areas there are a number of people who are in a position to help and it is usually a matter of making a couple of telephone calls to make contact with a counsellor or advisor. It is much wiser to contact some-one for advice rather than worry on your own about a problem.

The same people may be able to help if your concerns are about someone else who drinks too much or takes drugs. If you have a relative, a partner or a friend whose drinking or drug use is upsetting you, a professional will offer you advice about how *you* can cope with the situation. There is no need to fear that the professional will rush off to confront the drinker or drug user, and thereby get you into trouble. If this is your concern, then all you need to do is make your wishes clear to the professional at the start. Explain that it is you who would like advice and that it would cause additional problems for you if the drinker or drug user were contacted in any way. An agreement to this effect will set your mind at rest.

Local services vary enormously, and the task is to find out what is available in your area. Amongst those who can advise you are your own doctor, the student counselling service, the nurse or doctor in your school or occupational health department, the Citizen's Advice Bureau, the social services department and the Samaritans. You could also look in the telephone directory under 'alcohol' or 'drugs'. Here you are likely to find the telephone number of your nearest Alcohol or Drug Advice Centre, Alcoholics Anonymous contact, and private alcohol treatment facility.

All of the people mentioned above will have some knowledge of local counsellors, intervention facilities and support groups. You may be passed by one person to another, but do not be put off by this. The intention is not to fob you off, but to put you in touch with the most suitable counsellor or advisor.

Other readers who may be interested in further information are those who wish to organize education, training, or counselling for people with whom they work. These may be school teachers, personnel officers, counsellors, social workers, nurses or doctors. Professionals such as these may contact a number of organizations for advice at the addresses listed below.

Alcohol Concern
305 Grays Inn Road
London WC1X 8QF

Alcoholics Anonymous
PO Box 1
Stonebow House
Stonebow
York YO1 2NJ

Health Education Authority
Hamilton House
Mabledon Place
London WC1H 9TX

Scottish Council on Alcohol
137–145 Sauchiehall Street
Glasgow G2 4EW

Standing Conference on Drug Abuse
1–4 Hatton Place
Hatton Garden
London EC1N 8ND

The Advisory Council on Alcohol and Drug Education
1 Hulme Place
The Crescent
Salford
Greater Manchester M5 4QA

References

Abrams, D.B. and Niaura, R.S. (1987) 'Social learning theory', in Blane, H.T. and Leonard, K.E. (Eds) *Psychological Theories of Drinking and Alcoholism*, New York, The Guilford Press.

American Psychiatric Association (1952) *Diagnostic and Statistical Manual of Mental Disorders*, 1st ed., Washington DC, Author.

American Psychiatric Association (1968) *Diagnostic and Statistical Manual of Mental Disorders*, 2nd ed., Washington DC, Author.

American Psychiatric Association (1980) *Diagnostic and Statistical Manual of Mental Disorders*, 3rd ed., Washington DC, Author.

American Psychiatric Association (1987) *Diagnostic and Statistical Manual of Mental Disorders*, revised 3rd ed., Washington DC, Author.

Andersson, T. and Magnusson, D. (1988) 'Drinking habits and alcohol abuse among young men: A prospective longitudinal study', *Journal of Studies on Alcohol*, **49**, 245–52.

Armor, D.J. (1980) 'The Rand Reports and the analysis of relapse', in Edwards, G. and Grant, M. (Eds) *Alcoholism Treatment in Transition*, London, Croom Helm.

Arnett, J. (1992) 'Reckless behavior in adolescence: A developmental perspective', *Developmental Review*, **12**, 339–73.

Ashton, H. and Stepney, R. (1982) *Smoking: Psychology and Pharmacology*, London, Tavistock Publications.

Atkinson, R.L., Atkinson, R.C., Smith, E.E. and Bem, D.J. (1993) *Introduction to Psychology*, 11th ed., Fort Worth, TX, Harcourt Brace Jovanovich, Publishers.

Baer, J.S., Kivlahan, D.R., Fromme, K. and Marlatt, G.A. (1991) 'Secondary prevention of alcohol abuse with college student populations: A skills-training approach', in Heather, N., Miller, W.R. and Greeley, J. (Eds) *Self-Control and the Addictive Behaviours*, Botany, NSW Australia, Maxwell Macmillan Publishing Australia.

BAER, P.E., GARMEZY, L.B., McLAUGHLIN, R.J., POKORNY, A.D. and Wernick, M.J. (1987) 'Stress, coping, family conflict, and adolescent alcohol use', *Journal of Behavioral Medicine*, **10**, 449–66.

BANDURA, A. (1977a) *Social Learning Theory*, New York, Prentice Hall.

BANDURA, A. (1977b) 'Self-efficacy: Towards a unifying theory of behaviour change', *Psychological Review*, **84**, 191–215.

BENSLEY, L.S. and WU, R. (1991) 'The role of psychological reactance in drinking following alcohol prevention measures', *Journal of Applied Social Psychology*, **24**, 1111–24.

BERRIDGE, V. (1977) 'Opium and the historical perspective', *The Lancet*, 9 July, 78–80.

BERRIDGE, V. (1979) 'Morality and medical science: Concepts of narcotic addiction in Britain, 1820–1926', *Annals of Science*, **36**, 67–85.

BIEN, T.H., MILLER, W.R. and TONIGAN, J.S. (1993) 'Brief interventions for alcohol problems: A review', *Addiction*, **88**, 315–36.

BREWER, C. (1990) 'Combining pharmacological antagonists and behavioural psychotherapy in treating addictions: Why it is effective but unpopular', *British Journal of Psychiatry*, **157**, 34–40.

BRIGHAM, T. (1982) 'Self-management: A radical behavioural perspective', in KAROLY, P. and KANFER, F.H. (Eds) *Self-Management and Behavior Change: From Theory to Practice*. New York, Pergamon Press.

BROOK, J.S., WHITEMAN, M., GORDON, A.S., NOMURA, C. and BROOK, D.W. (1986) 'Onset of adolescent drinking: A longitudinal study of intrapersonal and interpersonal antecedents', *Advances in Alcohol and Substance Abuse*, **5**, 91–110.

BROOK, J.S., WHITEMAN, M., GORDON, A.S. and COHEN, P. (1989) 'Changes in drug involvement: A longitudinal study of childhood and adolescent determinants', *Psychological Reports*, **65**, 707–26.

BRY, B.H., McKEON, P. and PANDINA, R.J. (1982) 'Extent of drug use as a function of number of risk factors', *Journal of Abnormal Psychology*, **91**, 273–9.

CHANEY, E.F. (1989) 'Social skills training', in HESTER, R.K. and MILLER, W.R. (Eds) *Handbook of Alcoholism Treatment Approaches*, New York, Pergamon Press.

CHANEY, E.F., O'LEARY, M.R. and MARLATT, G.A. (1978) 'Skill training with alcoholics', *Journal of Consulting and Clinical Psychology*, **46**, 1092–104.

CHILDRESS, A.R., McLELLAN, A.T. and O'BRIEN, C.P. (1986) 'Abstinent opiate abusers exhibit conditioned craving, conditioned withdrawal and reductions in both through extinction', *British Journal of Addiction*, **81**, 655–60.

CHRISTIANSEN, B.A., GOLDMAN, M.S. and INN, A. (1982) 'Development of alcohol-related expectancies in adolescents: Separating pharmacological from social learning influences', *Journal of Consulting and Clinical Psychology*, **50**, 336–44.

CHRISTIANSEN, B.A., SMITH, G.T., ROEHLING, P.V. and GOLDMAN, S. (1989) 'Using alcohol expectancies to predict adolescent drinking behavior after one year', *Journal of Consulting and Clinical Psychology*, **57**, 93–99.

CLONINGER, C.R. (1987) 'Neurogenetic adaptive mechanisms in alcoholism', *Science*, **236**, 410–6.

COCHRANE, R. (1984) 'Social aspects of illegal drug use', in SANGER, D.J. and BLACKMAN, D.E. (Eds) *Aspects of Psychopharmacology*, London, Methuen.

COLE, G.D.H. and POSTGATE, R. (1971) *The Common People 1746–1946*, London, Methuen.

CONRAD, K.M., FLAY, B.R. and HILL, D. (1992) 'Why children start smoking cigarettes: Predictors of onset', *British Journal of Addiction*, **87**, 1711–24.

COOK, C.C.H. and GURLING, H.M.D. (1990) 'The genetic aspects of alcoholism and substance abuse: A review', in EDWARDS, G. and LADER, M. (Eds) *The Nature of Dependence*, Oxford, Oxford University Press.

COOPER, M.L., RUSSELL, M. and GEORGE, W.H. (1988) 'Coping, expectancies, and alcohol abuse: A test of social learning formulations', *Journal of Abnormal Psychology*, **97**, 218–30.

CRAIG, R.J. (1993) 'Contemporary trends in substance abuse', *Professional Psychology: Research and Practice*, **24**, 182–9.

CRAWFORD, G.A., WASHINGTON, M.C. and SENAY, E.C. (1983) 'Careers with heroin', *International Journal of the Addictions*, **18**, 701–15.

CYNN, V.E.H. (1992) 'Persistence and problem-solving skills in young male alcoholics', *Journal of Studies on Alcohol*, **53**, 57–62.

DARKES, J. and GOLDMAN, M.S. (1993) 'Expectancy challenge and drinking reduction: Experimental evidence for a mediational process', *Journal of Consulting and Clinical Psychology*, **61**, 344–53.

DAVIES, D.L. (1962) 'Normal drinking in recovered alcohol addicts', *Quarterly Journal of Studies on Alcohol*, **23**, 94–104.

DAVIES, J.B. (1992) *The Myth of Addiction*, Chur, Switzerland, Harwood Academic Publishers.

DAVIS, J.R. and TUNKS, E. (1991) 'Environments and addiction: A proposed taxonomy', *International Journal of the Addictions*, **25**, 805–26.

DE QUINCEY, T. (1907) *Confessions of an English Opium Eater*, London, J.M. Dent and Sons, Ltd.

DONOVAN, D.M. and CHANEY, E.F. (1985) 'Alcoholic relapse prevention and intervention: Models and methods', in MARLATT, G.A. and GORDON, J.R. (Eds) *Relapse Prevention*, New York, The Guilford Press.

DONOVAN, J.E., JESSOR, R. and COSTA, F.M. (1991) 'Adolescent health behavior and conventionality–unconventionality: An extension of problem behavior theory', *Health Psychology*, **10**, 52–61.

DOWNS, W.R. (1987) 'A panel study of normative structure, adolescent alcohol use, and peer alcohol use', *Journal of Studies on Alcohol*, **48**, 167–75.

D'ZURILLA, T.J. and GOLDFRIED, M.R. (1971) 'Problem solving and behavior modification', *Journal of Abnormal Psychology*, **78**, 107–26.

EDWARDS, G. and GROSS, M.M. (1976) 'Alcohol dependence: Provisional description of a clinical syndrome', *British Medical Journal*, **1**, 1058–61.

ELKINS, R.L. (1980) 'Covert sensitization treatment of alcoholism: Contributions of successful conditioning to subsequent abstinence maintenance', *Addictive Behaviors*, **5**, 67–89.

ELKINS, R.L. (1991) 'An appraisal of chemical aversion (emetic therapy) approaches to alcoholism treatment', *Behavior Research and Therapy*, **29**, 387–413.

ELLIOTT, D.S., HUIZINGA, D. and AGETON, A.S. (1985) *Explaining Delinquency and Drug Use*, Newbury Park, CA, Sage Publications.

FACULTY OF PUBLIC HEALTH MEDICINE, THE ROYAL COLLEGE OF PHYSICIANS (1991) *Alcohol and the Public Health*, Basingstoke, Macmillan.

FARRELL, A.D., DANISH, S.J. and HOWARD, C.W. (1992) 'Risk factors for drug use in urban adolescents: Identification and cross-validation', *American Journal of Community Psychology*, **20**, 263–86.

FINGARETTE, H. (1989) *Heavy Drinking: The Myth of Alcoholism as a Disease*, Berkeley, CA, University of California Press.

FRISCHER, M. and ELLIOTT, L. (1993) 'Discriminating needle exchange attenders from non-attenders', *Addiction*, **88**, 681–7.

GHODSE, H. (1989) *Drugs and Addictive Behaviour: A Guide to Treatment*, Oxford, Blackwell Scientific Publications.

GODDARD, E. and IKIN, C. (1989) *Drinking in England and Wales in 1987*, OPCS Social Survey Division, London, HMSO.

GOLDMAN, M.S. (1989) 'Alcohol expectancies as cognitive–behavioural psychology', in LOBERG, T., MILLER,W.R., NATHAN, P.E. and MARLATT, G.A. (Eds) *Addictive Behaviors: Prevention and Early Intervention*, Amsterdam, Swets and Zeitlinger.

GOLDMAN, M.S., BROWN, S.A. and CHRISTIANSEN, B.A. (1987) 'Expectancy theory: Thinking about drinking', in BLANE, H.T. and LEONARD, K.E.

(Eds) *Psychological Theories of Drinking and Alcoholism*. New York, The Guilford Press.

GOLDMAN, M.S., CHRISTIANSEN, B.A. and BROWN, S.A. (1987) *Alcohol Expectancy Questionnaire – Adolescent Form*, Odessa, FL, Psychological Assessment Resources Inc.

GOSSOP, M. (1982) *Living with Drugs*, London, Temple Smith.

GOSSOP, M. (1990) 'Compulsion, craving, and conflict', in WARBURTON, D.M. (Ed.) *Addiction Controversies*, Chur, Switzerland, Harwood Academic Publishers.

GOSSOP, M. (1993) 'Volatile substances and the law', *Addiction*, **88**, 311–4.

GOSSOP, M. and GRANT, M. (1991) 'A six country survey of the content and structure of heroin treatment programmes using methadone', *British Journal of Addiction*, **86**, 1151–60.

GRANT, B.F., HARFORD, T.C. and GRIGSON, M.B. (1988) 'Stability of alcohol consumption among youth: A national longitudinal survey', *Journal of Studies on Alcohol*, **49**, 253–60.

GUARDIAN (1993) 'Jailed drug users get tablets to clean needles', 30 October, p. 5.

HAWKINS, J.D., CATALANO, R.F. and MILLER, J.Y. (1992) 'Risk and protective factors for alcohol and other drug problems in adolescence and early adulthood: Implications for substance abuse prevention', *Psychological Bulletin*, **112**, 64–105.

HAWKS, D. (1991) 'Prevention and the locus of control: Internal, external, or somewhere in between?' in HEATHER, N., MILLER, W.R. and GREELEY, J. (Eds) *Self-Control and the Addictive Behaviours*, Botany, NSW Australia, Maxwell Macmillan Publishing Australia.

HEATHER, N. (1991) 'Impaired control over alcohol consumption', in HEATHER, N., MILLER, W.R. and GREELEY, J. (Eds) *Self-Control and the Addictive Behaviours*, Botany, NSW, Australia, Maxwell Macmillan Publishing Australia.

HEATHER, N. and ROBERTSON, I. (1981) *Controlled Drinking*, London, Methuen.

HEATHER, N. and ROBERTSON, I. (1985) *Problem Drinking: The New Approach*, Harmondsworth, Penguin.

HEATHER, N. and STALLARD, A. (1989) 'Does the Marlatt model underestimate the importance of conditioned craving in the relapse process?' in GOSSOP, M. (Ed.) *Relapse and Addictive Behaviour*, London, Tavistock/Routledge.

HEATHER, N., WHITTON, B. and ROBERTSON, I. (1986) 'Evaluation of a self-help manual for media-recruited problem drinkers: Six month follow-up results', *British Journal of Clinical Psychology*, **25**, 19–34.

HERBERT, M. (1987) *Conduct Disorders of Childhood and Adolescence: A Social Learning Perspective*, 2nd ed., Chichester, Wiley.

HODGSON, R.J. (1990) 'Cognitions and desire', in WARBURTON, D.M. (Ed.) *Addiction Controversies*, Chur, Switzerland, Harwood Academic Publishers.

HOPE, T. (1985) 'Drinking and disorder in the inner city', in *Implementing Crime Prevention Measures*, Home Office Research Study, No. 86, London, HMSO.

HOPKINS, R.H., MAUSS, A.L., KEARNEY, K.A. and WEISHEIT, R.A. (1988) 'Comprehensive evaluation of a model alcohol education curriculum', *Journal of Studies on Alcohol*, **49**, 38–50.

HOWARD, G. (1990) 'Some legal issues relating to passive smoking at the workplace', *British Journal of Addiction*, **85**, 873–82.

JELLINEK, E.M. (1952) 'Phases of alcohol addiction', *Quarterly Journal of Studies on Alcohol*, **13**, 673–84.

JELLINEK, E.M. (1960) *The Disease Concept of Alcoholism*, New Haven, CT, Hillhouse Press.

JESSOR, R. (1987) 'Problem behavior theory, psychosocial development, and adolescent problem drinking', *British Journal of Addiction*, **82**, 331–42.

JESSOR, R. (1992) 'Risk behavior in adolescence: A psychosocial framework for understanding action', *Developmental Review*, **12**, 374–90.

JESSOR, R. and JESSOR, S.L. (1977) *Problem Behavior and Psychosocial Development: A Longitudinal Study of Youth*, New York, Academic Press.

JOHNSON, V. (1988) 'Adolescent alcohol and marijuana use: A longitudinal assessment of a social learning perspective', *American Journal of Drug and Alcohol Abuse*, **14**, 419–39.

JOSEPHS, R.A. and STEELE, C.M. (1990) 'The two faces of alcohol myopia: Attentional mediation of psychological stress, *Journal of Abnormal Psychology*, **99**, 115–26.

KANDEL, D.B. (1985) 'On processes of peer influences in adolescent drug use: A developmental perspective', *Advances in Alcohol and Substance Use*, **4**, 139–63.

KANDEL, D.B., KESSLER, R.C. and MARGULIES, R.Z. (1978) 'Antecedents of adolescent initiation into stages of drug use: A developmental analysis', *Journal of Youth and Adolescence*, **7**, 13–40.

KANDEL, D.B. and RAVEIS, V.H. (1989) 'Cessation of illicit drug use in young adulthood', *Archives of General Psychiatry*, **46**, 109–16.

KANFER, F.H. and GAELICK, L. (1986) 'Self-management methods', in KANFER, F.H. and GOLDSTEIN, A.P. (Eds) *Helping People Change: A Textbook of Methods*, New York: Pergamon Press.

KEENE, J., STIMSON, G.V., JONES, S. and PARRY-LANGDON, N. (1993) 'Evaluation of syringe-exchange for HIV prevention among injecting drug users in rural and urban areas of Wales', *Addiction*, **88**, 1063–70.

KELLER, M. (1976) 'Problems with alcohol: An historical perspective', in FILSTEAD, W.J., ROSSI, J.J. and KELLER, M. (Eds) *Alcohol and Alcohol Problems*, Cambridge, MA, Ballinger Publishing Company.

KINDER, B.N., PAPE, N.E. and WALFISH, S. (1980) 'Drug and alcohol education programs: A review of outcome studies', *International Journal of the Addictions*, **15**, 1035–54.

KLEBER, H.D. (1989) 'Treatment of drug dependence: What works', *International Review of Psychiatry*, **1**, 81–100.

KLESGES, R.C., CIGRANG, J. and GLASGOW, R.E. (1987) 'Worksite smoking modification programs: A state-of-the-art review and directions for future research', *Current Psychological Research and Reviews*, **6**, 26–56.

KOHN, M. (1987) *Narcomania*, London, Faber and Faber.

KOZLOWSKI, L.T. and WILKINSON, D.A. (1987) 'Use and misuse of the concept of craving by alcohol, tobacco and drug researchers', *British Journal of Addiction*, **82**, 31–36.

KRAMER, M. (1988) 'Historical roots and structural bases of the International Classification of Diseases', in MEZZICH, J.E. and VON CRANACH, M. (Eds) *International Classification in Psychiatry*, Cambridge, Cambridge University Press.

KUMPFER, K.L. and TURNER, C.W. (1990) 'The social ecology model of adolescent substance abuse: Implications for prevention', *International Journal of the Addictions*, **25**, 435–63.

LEIGH, B.C. (1989) 'In search of the seven dwarves: Issues of measurement and meaning in alcohol expectancy research', *Psychological Bulletin*, **105**, 361–73.

LEX, B.W. (1991) 'Some gender differences in alcohol and polysubstance users', *Health Psychology*, **10**, 121–32.

LONGMATE, N. (1968) *The Water Drinkers*, London, Hamish Hamilton.

MACCOUN, R.J. (1993) 'Drugs and the law: A psychological analysis of drug prohibition', *Psychological Bulletin*, **113**, 497–512.

McKAY, J.R., MURPHY, R.T., RIVINUS, T.R. and MAISTO, S.A. (1991) 'Family dysfunction and alcohol and drug use in adolescent psychiatric inpatients', *Journal of the American Academy of Child and Adolescent Psychiatry*, **30**, 967–72.

McKECHNIE, R. (1985) 'Alcohol, contexts, and undesirable consequences: What is to be prevented?' in HEATHER, N., ROBERTSON, I. and DAVIES, P. (Eds) *The Misuse of Alcohol: Crucial Issues in Dependence, Treatment, and Prevention*, London, Croom Helm.

McLachlan, J.F.C. (1972) 'Benefit from group therapy as a function of patient–therapist match on conceptual level', *Psychotherapy: Theory, Research and Practice*, **9**, 317–23.

McMurran, M. and Hollin, C.R. (1993) *Young Offenders and Alcohol-Related Crime: A Practitioner's Guidebook*, Chichester, Wiley.

Madden, J.S. (1984) *A Guide to Alcohol and Drug Dependence*, Bristol, Wright.

Mahoney, M.J. and Thoresen, C.E. (1974) *Self-Control: Power to the Person*, Monterey, CA, Brookes/Cole.

Marks, J. (1991) 'The practice of controlled availability of illicit drugs', in Heather, N., Miller, W.R. and Greeley, J. (Eds) *Self-Control and the Addictive Behaviours*, Botany, NSW, Australia, Maxwell Macmillan Publishing Australia.

Marlatt, G.A. (1985a) 'Relapse prevention: Theoretical rationale and overview of the model', in Marlatt, G.A. and Gordon, J.R. (Eds) *Relapse Prevention*, New York, The Guilford Press.

Marlatt, G.A. (1985b) 'Situational determinants of relapse and skill-training interventions', in Marlatt, G.A. and Gordon, J.R. (Eds) *Relapse Prevention*, New York, The Guilford Press.

Marlatt, G.A. (1985c) 'Cognitive assessment and intervention procedures', in Marlatt, G.A. and Gordon, J.R. (Eds) *Relapse Prevention*, New York, The Guilford Press.

Marlatt, G.A., Demming, B. and Reid, J.B. (1973) 'Loss of control drinking in alcoholics: An experimental analogue', *Journal of Abnormal Psychology*, **81**, 233–41.

Marsh, A., Dobbs, J. and White, A. (1986) *Adolescent Drinking*, OPCS Social Survey Division, London, HMSO.

Marshall, E.J. (1990) 'The genetics of alcoholism', *British Journal of Hospital Medicine*, **44**, 317.

Mattick, R.P. and Heather, N. (1993) 'Developments in cognitive and behavioural approaches to substance misuse', *Current Opinion in Psychiatry*, **6**, 424–9.

May, C. (1993) 'Resistance to peer group pressure: An inadequate basis for alcohol education', *Health Education Research, Theory, and Practice*, **8**, 159–65.

Maynard, A. (1985) 'The role of economic measures in preventing drinking problems', in Heather, N., Robertson, I. and Davies, P. (Eds) *The Misuse of Alcohol: Crucial Issues in Dependence, Treatment, and Prevention*, London, Croom Helm.

Merry, J. (1966) 'The "loss of control" myth', *Lancet*, **4**, 1257–8.

Midanik, L.T., Klatsky, A.L. and Armstrong, M.A. (1990) 'Changes in drinking behavior: Demographic, psychosocial, and biomedical factors', *International Journal of the Addictions*, **25**, 599–619.

MILLER, W.R. (1978) 'Behavioral treatment of problem drinkers: A comparative outcome study of three controlled drinking therapies', *Journal of Consulting and Clinical Psychology*, **46**, 74–86.

MILLER, W.R. (1983) 'Motivational interviewing with problem drinkers', *Behavioural Psychotherapy*, **11**, 147–72.

MILLER, W.R. (1989) 'Matching individuals with interventions', in HESTER, R.K. and MILLER, W.R. (Eds) *Handbook of Alcoholism Treatment Approaches*, New York, Pergamon Press.

MILLER, W.R. and BACA, L.M. (1983) 'Two-year follow-up of bibliotherapy and therapist-directed controlled drinking training for problem drinkers', *Behavior Therapy*, **14**, 441–8.

MILLER, W.R. and BROWN, J.M. (1991) 'Self-regulation as a conceptual basis for the prevention and treatment of addictive behaviours', in HEATHER, N., MILLER, W.R. and GREELEY, J. (Eds) *Self-Control and the Addictive Behaviours*, Botany, NSW, Australia, Maxwell Macmillan Publishing Australia.

MILLER, W.R. and HESTER, R.K. (1986) 'The effectiveness of alcoholism treatment: What research reveals', in MILLER, W.R. and HEATHER, N. (Eds) *Treating Addictive Behaviors: Processes of Change*, New York, Plenum Press.

MILLER, W.R. and HESTER, R.K. (1989) 'Treating alcohol problems: Toward an informed eclecticism', in HESTER, R.K. and MILLER, W.R. (1989) *Handbook of Alcoholism Treatment Approaches*, New York, Pergamon Press.

MILLER, W.R., PECHACHEK, T.F. and HAMBURG, S. (1981) 'Group behavior therapy for problem drinkers', *International Journal of the Addictions*, **16**, 829–39.

MILLER, W.R. and ROLLNICK, S. (1991) *Motivational Interviewing: Preparing People to Change Addictive Behavior*, New York, The Guilford Press.

MILLER, W.R. and SOVEREIGN, R.G. (1989) 'The Check-Up: A model for early intervention in addictive behaviors', in LOBERG, T., MILLER, W.R., NATHAN, P.E. and MARLATT, G.A. (Eds) *Addictive Behaviors: Prevention and Early Intervention*, Amsterdam, Swets and Zeitlinger.

MILLER, W.R. and TAYLOR, C.A. (1980) 'Relative effectiveness of bibliotherapy, individual, and group self-control training in the treatment of problem drinkers', *Addictive behaviors*, **5**, 13–24.

MONTI, P.M., ABRAMS, D.B., KADDEN, R.M. and COONEY, N.L. (1989) *Treating Alcohol Dependence*, London, Cassell.

MUSTO, D.F. (1973) *The American Disease: Origins of Narcotic Control*, New Haven, Yale University Press.

NADELMANN, E.A. (1988) 'US drug policy: A bad export', *Foreign Policy*, **70**, 83–107.

NADELMANN, E.A. (1989) 'Drug prohibition in the United States: Costs, consequences, and alternatives', *Science*, **245**, 939–47.

NADELMANN, E.A. (1992) 'Thinking seriously about alternatives to drug prohibition', *Daedalus*, **121**, 85–132.

NATHAN, P.E. (1988) 'The addictive personality is the behavior of the addict', *Journal of Consulting and Clinical Psychology*, **56**, 183–8.

NATHAN, P.E. (1991) 'Substance use disorders in the DSM-IV', *Journal of Abnormal Psychology*, **100**, 356–61.

NEWCOMB, M.D. and BENTLER, P.M. (1989) 'Substance use and abuse among children and teenagers', *American Psychologist*, **44**, 242–8.

NEWCOMB, M.D., MADDAHIAN, E. and BENTLER, P.M. (1986) 'Risk factors for drug use among adolescents: Concurrent and longitudinal analyses', *American Journal of Public Health*, **76**, 525–31.

O'CONNOR, J. (1990) 'Mass media and the prevention of drug problems: A psychological appraisal', *Drug and Alcohol Review*, **9**, 177–85.

OETTING, E.R. (1992) 'Planning programs for prevention of deviant behavior: A psychosocial model', in TRIMBLE, J., BOLEK, C. and MIEMCRYK, S. (Eds) *Ethnic and Multi-Cultural Drug Abuse*, Binghamton, NY, Harrington Park Press.

O'FARRELL, T.J., CUTTER, H.S.G., CHOQUETTE, K.A., FLOYD, F.J. and BAYOG, R.D. (1992) 'Behavioral marital therapy for male alcoholics: Marital and drinking adjustment during the two years after treatment', *Behavior Therapy*, **23**, 529–49.

ORFORD, J. (1985) *Excessive Appetites: A Psychological View of Addictions*, Chichester, Wiley.

PAREDES, A. (1976) 'The history of the concept of alcoholism', in TARTER, R.E. and SUGERMAN, A.A. (Eds) *Alcoholism*, Reading, MA, Addison Wesley.

PARSONS, O.A. (1989) 'Impairment in sober alcoholics' cognitive functioning: The search for determinants', in LOBERG, T., MILLER, W.R., NATHAN, P.E. and MARLATT, G.A. (Eds) *Addictive Behaviors: Prevention and Early Intervention*, Amsterdam, Swets and Zeitlinger.

PARSSINEN, T.M. (1983) *Secret Passions, Secret Remedies: Narcotic Drugs in British Society 1820–1930*. Philadelphia, PA, Institute for the Study of Human Issues Inc.

PEELE, S. (1985) *The Meaning of Addiction*, Lexington, MA, D.C. Heath and Company.

PLANT, M.A. (1987) *Drugs in Perspective*, London, Hodder and Stoughton.

POLICH, J.M. (1980) 'Patterns of remission in alcoholism', in EDWARDS, G. and GRANT, M. (Eds) *Alcoholism Treatment in Transition*, London, Croom Helm.

POMERLEAU, O.F., FERTIG, J., BAKER, L. and COONEY, N. (1983) 'Reactivity to alcohol cues in alcoholics and non-alcoholics: Implications for a stimulus control analysis of drinking', *Addictive Behaviors*, **8**, 1–10.

PROCHASKA, J.O., DiCLEMENTE, C.C. and NORCROSS, J.C. (1992) 'In search of how people change: Applications to addictive behaviors', *American Psychologist*, **47**, 1102–14.

RACHLIN, H. (1970) *Introduction to Modern Behaviorism*, San Francisco, W.H. Freeman.

RAMSAY, M. (1982) *City Centre Crime: The Scope for Situational Prevention*, Research and Planning Unit Paper, No. 10, London, Home Office.

RANKIN, H., HODGSON, R. and STOCKWELL, T. (1979) 'The concept of craving and its measurement', *Behavior Research and Therapy*, **17**, 389–96.

RHODES, J.E. and JASON, L.A. (1988) *Preventing Substance Abuse Among Children and Adolescents*, New York, Pergamon Press.

ROBINS, L.N., HELZER, J.E. and DAVIS, D.H. (1975) 'Narcotic use in southeast Asia and afterward', *Archives of General Psychiatry*, **32**, 955–61.

ROHSENOW, D.J., NIAURA, R.S., CHILDRESS, A.R., ABRAMS, D.B. and MONTI, P.M. (1991) 'Cue reactivity in addictive behaviors: Theoretical and treatment implications', *International Journal of the Addictions*, **25**, 957–93.

ROHSENOW, D.J., SMITH, R.E. and JOHNSON, J. (1986) 'Stress management as a prevention program for heavy social drinkers', *Addictive Behaviors*, **10**, 45–54.

ROOM, R. and GREENFIELD, T. (1993) 'Alcoholics Anonymous, other 12-step movements and psychotherapy in the US population, 1990', *Addiction*, **88**, 555–62.

ROSE, S., LEWONTIN, R.C. and KAMIN, L.J. (1984) *Not in Our Genes: Biology, Ideology, and Human Nature*, Harmondsworth, Penguin Books.

ROSENBERG, H. (1993) 'Prediction of controlled drinking by alcoholics and problem drinkers', *Psychological Bulletin*, **113**, 129–39.

RUNDALL, T.G. and BRUVOLD, W.H. (1988) 'A meta-analysis of school-based smoking and alcohol use prevention programs', *Health Education Quarterly*, **15**, 317–34.

SAUNDERS, B. (1985) 'The case for controlling alcohol consumption', in HEATHER, N., ROBERTSON, I. and DAVIES, P. (Eds) *The Misuse of*

Alcohol: Crucial Issues in Dependence, Treatment, and Prevention, London: Croom Helm.

SAUNDERS, B. and ALLSOP, S. (1991) 'Incentives and restraints: Clinical research into problem drug use and self-control', in HEATHER, N., MILLER, W.R. and GREELEY, J. (Eds) *Self-Control and the Addictive Behaviours*, Botany, NSW, Australia, Maxwell Macmillan Publishing Australia.

SHAW, S. (1979) 'A critique of the concept of the alcohol dependence syndrome', *British Journal of Addiction*, **74**, 339–48.

SHAW, S. (1982) 'What is problem drinking?' in PLANT, M.A. (Ed.) *Drinking and Problem Drinking*, London, Junction Books.

SHIPLEY, T.E. (1987) 'Opponent process theory', in BLANE, H.T. and LEONARD, K.E. (Eds) *Psychological Theories of Drinking and Alcoholism*, New York, The Guilford Press.

SIEGEL, S. (1988) 'Drug anticipation and drug tolerance', in LADER, M. (Ed.) *The Psychopharmacology of Addiction*, Oxford, Oxford University Press.

SINGLE, E. (1993) 'The interaction between policy and research in the implementation of server training', *Addiction, (Supplement)*, **88**, 105S–13S.

SISSON, R.W. and AZRIN, N.H. (1989) 'The Community Reinforcement Approach', in HESTER, R.K. and MILLER, W.R. (Eds) *Handbook of Alcoholism Treatment Approaches*, New York, Pergamon.

SKIRROW, J. and SAWKA, E. (1987) 'Alcohol and drug abuse prevention strategies: An overview', *Contemporary Drug Problems*, Summer, 147–241.

SOLOMON, R.L. (1980) 'The opponent process theory of acquired motivation: The affective dynamics of addiction', *American Psychologist*, **35**, 691–712.

SPEAR, H.B. (1982) 'British experience in the management of opiate dependence', in GLATT, M.M. and MARKS, J. (Eds) *The Dependence Phenomenon*, Lancaster, MPT Press.

STALL, R. and BIERNACKI, P. (1986) 'Spontaneous remission from the problematic use of substances: An inductive model derived from a comparative analysis of the alcohol, opiate, tobacco, and food/obesity literature', *International Journal of the Addictions*, **21**, 1–23.

STIMSON, G.V. (1990) 'AIDS and HIV: The challenge for British drug services', *British Journal of Addiction*, **85**, 329–39.

STIMSON, G.V., DOLAN, K.A., DONOGHOE, M.C. and LART, R. (1989) 'The pilot syringe-exchange project in England and Scotland: A summary of the evaluation', *British Journal of Addiction*, **84**, 1283–4.

STOCKWELL, T. (1991) 'Experimental analogues of loss of control: A review of human drinking studies', in HEATHER, N., MILLER, W.R. and GREELEY, J. (Eds) *Self-Control and the Addictive Behaviours*, Botany, NSW, Australia, Maxwell Macmillan Publishing Australia.

STOCKWELL, T. and TOWN, C. (1989) 'Anxiety and stress management', in HESTER, R.K. and MILLER, W.R. (Eds) *Handbook of Alcoholism Treatment Approaches*, New York, Pergamon.

STRANG, J. (1990) 'Heroin and cocaine: New technologies, new problems', in WARBURTON, D.M. (Ed.) *Addiction Controversies*, Chur, Switzerland, Harwood Academic Publishers.

STUART, R.B. (1974) 'Teaching facts about drugs: Pushing or preventing?' *Journal of Educational Psychology*, **66**, 189–201.

SWADI, H. (1988) 'Drug and substance use among 3333 London adolescents', *British Journal of Addiction*, **83**, 935–42.

SWADI, H. and ZEITLIN, H. (1988) 'Peer influence and adolescent substance abuse: A promising side?' *British Journal of Addiction*, **83**, 153–7.

SZASZ, T. (1974) *Ceremonial Chemistry*, Garden City, NY, Anchor Press/Doubleday.

TARTER, R.E. (1988) 'Are there inherited behavioral traits that predispose to substance abuse?' *Journal of Consulting and Clinical Psychology*, **56**, 189–96.

TETHER, P. and ROBINSON, D. (1986) *Preventing Alcohol Problems: A Guide to Local Action*, London, Tavistock Publications.

THOMPSON, K.M. (1989) 'Effects of alcohol use on adolescents' relations with peers and self-esteem: Patterns over time', *Adolescence*, **24**, 837–49.

THORLEY, A. (1985) 'The role of mass media campaigns in alcohol health education', in HEATHER, N., ROBERTSON, I. and DAVIES P. (Eds) *The Misuse of Alcohol: Crucial Issues in Dependence, Treatment, and Prevention*, London, Croom Helm.

TOBER, G. (1991) 'Helping the pre-contemplator', in DAVIDSON, R., ROLLNICK, S. and MACEWAN, I. (Eds) *Counselling Problem Drinkers*, London, Tavistock/Routledge.

TOBLER, N.S. (1986) 'Meta-analysis of 143 adolescent drug prevention programs', *Journal of Drug Issues*, **16**, 537–67.

TOLMAN, E.G. (1932) *Purposive Behavior in Animals and Man*, New York, Appleton-Century-Crofts.

TUCHFELD, B.S. (1981) 'Spontaneous remission in alcoholics: Empirical observations and theoretical implications', *Journal of Studies on Alcohol*, **42**, 626–41.

TUCKER, J.A., VUCHINICH, R.E. and DOWNEY, K.K. (1992) 'Substance abuse', in TURNER, S.M., CALHOUN, K.S. and ADAMS H.E. (Eds) *Handbook of Clinical Behavior Therapy*, 2nd ed., New York, Wiley.

VAN HASSETT, V.B., HULL, J.A., KEMPTON, T., and BUKSTEIN, O.G., (1993) 'Social skills and depression in adolescent substance abusers', *Addictive Behaviors*, **18**, 9–18.

VELICER, W.F., DiCLEMENTE, C.C., ROSSI, J.S. and PROCHASKA, J.O. (1990) 'Relapse situations and self-efficacy: An integrative model', *Addictive Behaviors*, **15**, 271–83.

WARD, J., DARKE, S., HALL, W. and MATTICK, R. (1992) 'Methadone maintenance and the human immunodeficiency virus: Current issues in treatment and research', *British Journal of Addiction*, **87**, 447–53.

WEBB, J.A., BAER, P.E., FRANCIS, D.J. and CAID, C.D. (1993) 'Relationship among social and intrapersonal risk, alcohol expectancies, and alcohol usage among early adolescents, *Addictive Behaviors*, **8**, 127–34.

WEBB, J.A., BAER, P.E., McLAUGHLIN, R.J., McKELVEY, R.S. and CAID, C.D. (1991) 'Risk factors and their relation to initiation of alcohol use among early adolescents', *Journal of the American Academy of Child and Adolescent Psychiatry*, **30**, 563–8.

WERCH, C.E., GORMAN, D.R. and MARTY, P.J. (1987) 'Relationship between alcohol consumption and alcohol problems in young adults', *Journal of Drug Education*, **17**, 261–76.

WILDE, G.J.S. (1993) 'Effects of mass media communications on health and safety habits: An overview of issues and evidence', *Addiction*, **88**, 983–96.

WILKINSON, D.A. (1991) 'Addictive behaviours and the neuropsychology of self-control', in HEATHER, N., MILLER, W.R. and GREELEY, J. (Eds) *Self-Control and the Addictive Behaviours*, Botany, NSW, Australia, Maxwell Macmillan Publishing Australia.

WILSON, G.T. (1988) 'Alcohol and anxiety', *Behavior Research and Therapy*, **26**, 369–81.

WINDLE, M. (1991) 'The difficult temperament in adolescence: Associations with substance use, family support, and problem behaviors', *Journal of Clinical Psychology*, **47**, 310–15.

WISE, R.A. (1988) 'The neurobiology of craving: Implications for the understanding and treatment of addiction', *Journal of Abnormal Psychology*, **97**, 118–32.

WORLD HEALTH ORGANIZATION (1948) *Manual of the International Statistical Classification of Diseases, Injuries and Cause of Death (6th Revision)*, Geneva, World Health Organization.

WORLD HEALTH ORGANIZATION (1955) *Manual of the International Statistical Classification of Diseases, Injuries and Cause of Death (7th Revision)*, Geneva, World Health Organization.

WORLD HEALTH ORGANIZATION (1965) *Manual of the International Statistical Classification of Diseases, Injuries and Cause of Death (8th Revision)*, Geneva, World Health Organization.

WORLD HEALTH ORGANIZATION (1977) *Manual of the International Statistical Classification of Diseases, Injuries and Cause of Death (9th Revision)*, Geneva, World Health Organization.

YATES, A.J. (1990) 'The natural history of heroin addiction', in WARBURTON, D.M. (Ed.) *Addiction Controversies*, Chur, Switzerland, Harwood Academic Publishers.

YATES, F. and HEBBLETHWAITE, D. (1985) 'Using natural resources for preventing drinking problems', in HEATHER, N., ROBERTSON, I. and DAVIES, P. (Eds) *The Misuse of Alcohol: Crucial Issues in Dependence, Treatment, and Prevention*, London, Croom Helm.

YOUNG, R.M., OEI, T.P.S. and KNIGHT, R.G. (1990) 'The tension reduction hypothesis revisited: An alcohol expectancy perspective', *British Journal of Addiction*, **85**, 31–40.

ZACUNE, J. (1976) 'A comparison of Canadian narcotic addicts in Great Britain and Canada', in EDWARDS, G., RUSSELL, M.A.H., HAWKS, D. and MACCAFFERTY, M. (Eds) *Drugs and Drug Dependence*, Farnborough, Hants, Saxon House/Lexington Books.

ZUCKERMAN, M. (1979) *Sensation Seeking: Beyond the Optimal Level of Arousal*, Hillsdale, NJ, Erlbaum.

Index

'a' process 39–40
'A' state 39–40
AA 12–13, 128–9, 160
abstinence 13, 22–3, 104
abstinence violation effect 120
academic achievement as protective
    factor 68–9
addiction
  classification 19–21
  definition 1, 48–50
  genetic aspects 28, 80
  reversibility 13, 22–5, 47–8
addictive behaviours 49–50
  application of psychological theories
    to 34–45
  continuum of 46–7
  factors determining 31–4
  implications of psychological
    approach 45–8
  interaction of factors in 45–6
adolescence
  maintenance and progression of
    substance use 69–71
  prevalence of substance use 53–6
  protective factors 68–9
  risk factors of initiation 56–68
Adult Children of Alcoholics 128
advertising 142–3
advice services 159–60
Advisory Council on Alcohol and Drug
    Education 160
AEQ-A 64–5
affective contrast 39
affective habituation 39
affective withdrawal 39

age, and substance use 53–6
agenda-setting 143
AIDS 154
Al-Anon 128
Al-Ateen 128
alcohol
  attention narrowing effect 85–6
  controls on availability 133–5, 137–8
  licensing laws 134–5
  metabolic sensitivity to 33, 78–9
  priming dose 89
  taxation 135
  tension and stress reducing effects
    84–6
  withdrawal symptoms 83
alcohol abuse, differentiation from
    alcoholism 15
Alcohol Concern 160
alcohol dependence syndrome 18–19
Alcohol Expectancy Questionnaire –
    Adolescent Form 64–5
alcohol myopia 85–6
alcohol use
  and age 53–4
  and damage to central nervous system
    92
  expectancy factors 64–6
  harm minimization 152–4
  history of responses to 4–28
  legal aspects 57
  and life events 66, 67
  moderation or abstinence as goal
    104
  social function 51–2
  work place policies 145

Alcoholics Anonymous 12–13, 128–9, 160
alcoholism
  classic disease model 12–15
  classification 14, 79, 92
  differentiation from alcohol abuse 15
  origin of term 10
alpha alcoholism 14
American Temperance Society 6
amphetamines 17
anger in childhood 150
Antabuse 127
antidipsotropic drugs 127
antisocial behaviour 28
anxiety reduction by alcohol use 84–6
assertiveness skills 151
assessment methods 107
automatic processing 108
AVE 120
aversion therapy 40, 123–4

'b' process 39–40
'B' state 39–40
balanced placebo design 26–7
barbiturates 17
behaviour, factors determining 31–4
behavioural factors in initiation 61–4
Behavioural Self-Control Training
  107–11
behavioural skills as factor in behaviour
  32–3
benefits, pay-off against costs 76–8, 94
beta alcoholism 14
biological determinism 80
biopsychosocial model 46
Brain Committee 17
BSCT 107–11

cannabis 17
  decriminalization 31
careers of substance use 69–71
central nervous system, alcohol damage
  92
chaining 38
change 97–8
  by behavioural self-control training
    107–11
  by non-psychological interventions
    126–30
  by psychological interventions 104–26
  by skills training 111–17

and lifestyle modification 121–2
  motivation to 104–7
  processes of 102
  and relapse prevention 117–21
  stages of 100–1
  unassisted 98–100
Children and Young Persons (Protection
    from Tobacco) Act 1991 57
cigarette smoking
  in childhood and adolescence 54, 55
  legal aspects 57
  work place policies 146
civil liability 153
classical conditioning 34–6, 83
classification
  addiction 19–21
  alcoholism 14
  drugs 58
cocaine 15
coffee-drinking, social attitudes to 51
cognitive functioning and loss of control
    92–3, 95
cold turkey 126
community reinforcement 121–2
complex behaviours 38
conditioned response 34
conditioned stimulus 34
conditioning 25–7
*Confessions of an English Opium Eater,
    The* 7–8
confrontation 104
contemplation
  of change 100
  chronic 101
contingency management 36, 110
control, loss of 13, 21–2, 75, 86–95
  cognitive element 26–7
controlled processing 108
conventionality 43–4
cooperative learning 149
coping
  alcohol use as mechanism 84–5
  and loss of control 93
  with temptation 118–19
costs, pay-off against benefits 76–8, 94
covert modelling 119
covert sensitization 124
crack 52
craving 13, 22, 27, 87–92
  conditioned 35

cue exposure 123
  with response prevention 35
cue reactivity 88–92, 95
cultural determinism 80
cultural factors in behaviour 31–2

Dangerous Drugs Act 1920 15
Dangerous Drugs Regulations 1921 15
De Quincey, Thomas 7–8
decision review 118
decisional self-control 109–10
Defence of the Realm Act 1916 15
defensive strategies 95–6
definitions
  addiction 1, 48–50
  dependence 76
  drug 2–4
  drug abuse 4
delinquency, and initiation of substance
    use 61–4
delirium tremens 83
delta alcoholism 14
denial 96, 104
dependence 73–6, 94–6
  concept of 18–19
  definition 76
  and diminished control 86–94
  and excessive indulgence 76–86
  separation between physical and
    psychological 88
depression 28
designer drugs 52
desire 13, 22, 27, 35, 87–92
determinism 2
detoxification 126–7
deviant behaviour 43–4, 61–2
  model for prevention 147, 148
Diagnostic and Statistical Manual of
    Mental Disorders, classification of
    addiction 20
diary, self-monitoring 108, 109
dipsomania 10
discrimination 35–6
discrimination training 108
discriminative stimuli 38
disease model 2
  of alcoholism 12–15
  challenges to 21–8
  of drug addiction 15–18
  history of 9–11

dispositional tolerance 83
disulfiram 127
dopaminergic system 79
Drinker's Check-Up 107
drug abuse, definition 4
drug addiction, disease model 15–18
drug therapy 127–8
drug use
  and age 54–5
  costs and benefits 77–8
  harm minimization 154–5
  history of responses to 4–28
  legal aspects 58
  social function 52
  subcultures 81–2
drugs
  addictive 2, 3
  classification 58
  controls on availability 135–8
  defining 2–4
  exercise of control over 3
  legalization 31, 136–7
  psychoactive 3–4
DSM, classification of addiction in 20
DTs 83
Dunlop, John 6–7

Edwards, Griffith 18
emergency procedures 120
emotionality 80
endorphins 49
environmental factors in behaviour 32
epsilon alcoholism 14
excessive indulgence 76–86
expectancy challenge 124–5
expectancy factors 65, 66
expectancy theory 44–5
extinction 35, 38

family
  bonding to 59
  conflict within 59
  factors in behaviour 32
  harm minimization within 153–4
  influence relative to peer group 61
  influences on initiation 58–60
  management 59
  role in prevention 147–9
  support programmes 147–9
family therapy 122

feedback 112
feelings as factor in behaviour 33
Finland, controls on alcohol supply and consumption 134
flushing in response to alcohol 33
forethought 41
free will 1
frontal lobes, and control of behaviour 92
functional tolerance 83

gamma alcoholism 14
gender
    and substance use in adolescence 55
    and susceptibility to effects of alcohol 33
generalization 35–6, 38
genetic aspects of addiction 28, 80
goal setting 108–9, 113
goal violation effect 119–20
Gross, Milton M. 18
GVE 119–20

harm minimization 152–7
Harrison Act 1914 16
health education
    media-based 142–5
    school-based 139–42
Health Education Authority 160
heroin 15
    cues eliciting craving in addicts 90, 91
    registration of addicts 17
    similarities between addiction and work 81
history
    of disease model 9–11
    of responses to drug and alcohol use 4–28
HIV infection 48, 154, 156–7
hyperactivity 80

ICD, classification of addiction in 20–1
imagery 116
industrialization 5–6
inebriety 11–12
information services 159–60
initiation 52
    risk factors for 56–68
International Classification of Diseases, classification of addiction in 20–1

intervention
    behavioural self-control training 107–11
    goals of 103–4
    lifestyle modification 121–2
    matching to the client 98, 101–4
    modules 102–3
    motivational techniques 104–7
    non-psychological 126–30
    psychological 104–26
    relapse prevention 117–21
    skills training 111–17
    success of 97–8
    triadic model 149
interviewing, motivational 105–7

jazz, corrupting influence of 17
Jellinek, E.M. 13–15

Kerr, Norman 11
Kolb, Lawrence 16
Korsakoff's syndrome 154

lapses, coping with 119–20
laudanum 5
legal aspects of initiation 57–8
Levinstein, Eduard 10
licensed premises, and harm minimization 153
life events and alcohol use 66, 67
lifestyle
    as factor in behaviour 32
    modification 121–2
liver cirrhosis, mortality levels 133–4
Liverpool Temperance Society 6
Liversey, Joseph 7
lysergic acid diethylamide (LSD) 17

maintenance
    of change 100
    of substance use 52–3, 69–71
maintenance prescription 16, 17, 127, 154
marital therapy 122
matching hypothesis 101
maturing out 98
media, health education via 142–5
medical model *see* disease model
methadone 15, 127, 154
Misuse of Drugs Act 1971 58
Misuse of Drugs Regulations 1985 58

modelling 41, 112
  covert 119
  and initiation 59
moderation 74, 104
monomania 10
moral model 1–2
morphine 10–11
motivational intervention techniques
    104–7
motivational interviewing 105–7
muscle relaxation 116

naltrexone 127
nature-nurture argument 80
needle-exchange schemes 155
negative punishment 37
negative reinforcement 37, 40, 79
negative thinking 115
non-verbal skills 111

operant conditioning 36–9
opioids, withdrawal symptoms 83
opium
  consumption 5, 7–8
  smoking 8
  trade in 11–12
Opium War 11
opponent process theory 39–40
Oriental flushing 33
outcome expectancy 44–5, 64–6
  challenge 124–5

parents *see* family
partial reinforcement 38
passive smoking 145
Pavlov, Ivan 34
pay-off matrix 76
peer counsellors 142
peer group
  influence of 32, 60–1
  role in prevention 150
  selection 60
  and socialization 60
personality, addictive 27–8
Pharmacy Act 1868 8
physical factors in behaviour 33
PIG 118
positive punishment 37
positive reinforcement 37, 79
precontemplation stage in change 100

preparation for change 100
prevalence of substance use 53–6
prevention 131–2
  by changing culture and context
    138–46
  by controls on availability 132–8
  by strengthening individual resilience
    146–51
  and harm minimization 152–7
  psychosocial model 147, 148
priming dose 89
problem behaviour theory 43–4, 61–2,
    148
problem of immediate gratification 118
problem solving 93
  training 112–14
Prohibition 7, 12, 132–3
proneness to problem behaviour 43
protective factors 68–9
protracted self-control 110
psychiatric classification 19–21
psychoanalysis 16
psychological factors in initiation 64–8
psychological theories 34–45
  implications regarding addiction
    45–8
psychosocial proneness 43
psychotherapy 126
punishment 37

Rand Report 23–4
rate control 110
reactance 140–1
reactivity effect 108
reckless behaviours 63
refusal skills 151
rehabilitation 128
rehearsal 112
reinforcement 36–8, 40, 78–81, 94
relapse 89–90, 101
  coping with 119–20
  determinants 117
  prevention 117–21
  rehearsal 120
relaxation techniques 116
resilience, increasing 146–51
response prevention 123
risk
  concept of 43
  factors in initiation 56–68

graded practice in situations of
120–1
implications of 68–9
road traffic accidents, harm minimization
152
role-play 112
Rolleston Report 16
rule setting 109–10
Rush, Benjamin 9–10

school
health education in 139–42
role in prevention 149–50
Scottish Council on Alcohol 160
seemingly irrelevant decisions 118–19
self-change 98–100
self-control
capabilities required for 92
training in 107–11
self-efficacy 41–2, 93–4, 95
self-esteem 66
self-monitoring 108, 109
self-motivational statements 105
self-punishment 110
self-regulation 41, 94–5
self-report measures 53
self-reward 110
self-statements, positive 118
sensation seeking 63, 150
SIDs 118–19
skills training 111–17
Skinner, B.F. 36
social factors in behaviour 32
social learning theory 41–3
social norms 138–9
social skills training 111–12
Society for the Diffusion of Useful
Knowledge 7
Society for the Study of Inebriety 11
Society for Suppression of the Opium
Trade 12
solvent use, legal aspects 57–8
spontaneous recovery 35
spontaneous remission 98
Standing Conference on Drug Abuse
160
stimulus control 109–10

stress
management training 115–17
reduction by alcohol use 84–6
as risk factor for initiation 66, 67
subcultures of drug use 81–2
substance availability, controls on
132–8
substance dependence *see* dependence
substance use
careers 69–71
changing culture and context 138–46
developmental progression 62
and fashion 52
history of responses to 4–28
prevalence 53–6
risk factors for initiation 56–68
social function 51–2
symbolism 41

temperament
and dependence 80
and initiation of substance use 63–4
temperance movement 6–7
temptation, coping with 118–19
tension reduction by alcohol use 84–6
therapeutic communities 129–30
therapist, tasks 102
thoughts as factor in behaviour 33
tolerance 21, 25, 40, 82–3
town planning and harm minimization
152–3
triadic model of intervention 149
Trotter, Thomas 10
twelve-step programmes 128–9

unconditioned response 34
unconditioned stimulus 34
unconventionality 43–4, 63

verbal skills 111
Vietnam war, drug use by veterans 24
vitamin supplements 154
vulnerability, decreasing 146–51

withdrawal symptoms 21, 26, 82–3
work, similarities with addiction 81
work place policies 145–6